THE PARENT'S GUIDE TO

CHILDREN'S
CONGENITAL
HEART DEFECTS

D0965027

THE PARENT'S GUIDE TO

CHILDREN'S CONGENITAL HEART DEFECTS

What They Are, How to Treat Them, How to Cope with Them

Gerri Freid Kramer and **Shari Maurer**

Foreword by Sylvester Stallone and Jennifer Flavin-Stallone

THREE RIVERS PRESS · NEW YORK

The information contained in this book is not meant to diagnose or treat your child or to substitute for professional medical attention. Share this book with your doctor so you can work more effectively with him or her. Always consult your child's personal physician with any questions you may have.

Any quotes by parents reflect the opinions and knowledge of these parents and are not necessarily the opinions of the medical experts or the authors of this book.

Published by Three Rivers Press, New York, New York.
Member of the Crown Publishing Group.

Random House, Inc. New York, Toronto, London, Sydney, Auckland
www.randomhouse.com

THREE RIVERS PRESS is a registered trademark and the Three Rivers Press colophon is a trademark of Random House, Inc.

Printed in the United States of America

Design by Rhea Braunstein

Library of Congress Cataloging-in-Publication Data
Kramer, Gerri Freid.
The parent's guide to children's congenital heart defects : what they are, how to treat them, how to cope with them / Gerri Freid Kramer and Shari Maurer.—1st ed.
Includes bibliographical references.
1. Congenital heart disease in children—Treatment. 2. Heart—Diseases—Treatment. 3. Children—Diseases. 4. Consumer education. I. Maurer, Shari. II. Title.
RJ426.C64 K73 2001
618.92'12043—dc21
2001027785

ISBN 0-609-80775-7

10 9 8 7 6 5 4 3 2

FIRST EDITION

To Elisabeth and Max,
and in memory of our friend
Karin Newman Krueger

ACKNOWLEDGMENTS

∞

WE WOULD LIKE to thank everyone who has contributed to this book. First, thanks go to our team of medical experts. We are touched by how generously and enthusiastically they gave their time and expertise. And our sincere thanks go to the many parents who have added their thoughts to the book, whose personal experiences and advice will be invaluable to readers in similar situations. We weren't able to include quotes from all the many parents who contributed to this book, but the spirit of what they told us in surveys and interviews helped shape the book, and for that we are grateful.

As we were writing the book, we learned much from the parents who participate in the PD Heart Internet support group. Two moms in particular—Mona Barmash and Sue Dove—were of continual help to us. Their examples are inspirations to us all.

Scott Myers and the staff of Boggy Creek Camp in Orlando, Florida, and Ken Coulon of the Edward J. Madden Memorial Open Hearts Camp in Great Barrington, Massachusetts, were wonderful and opened up their camps to us so that we could not only see how valuable the camps are to children with CHD, but also speak with the children and their parents about how CHD has affected their lives. Similarly, we are grateful for the opportunity to learn from the moms in the support group at Morristown Memorial Hospital and hear about their concerns firsthand.

Many thanks to those who helped us at the many medical centers we worked with: Mary Barrington, Beth Bruton, and Coleen Miller at Duke; Barbara Capps at Vanderbilt, Donna Heller at Columbia, Wanda Kaminski at Morristown Memorial Hospital, Barbara Lefkowksi at Yale, Cheryl Metiaski at Baylor University, Tara O'Ryan at Brigham and Women's Hospital/Children's Hospital, Lynn Pappas at UCLA, Diane Rode at Mt. Sinai Medical Center, Cathy Rubenstein at Medical University of South Carolina, Connie Nixon at the University of Florida, and Angela Israel at the Pediatric Specialty Clinic in Roanoke, who also reviewed the book and provided ongoing support, and to all of the other people we spoke to during the creation of this book.

Thanks, too, to our doctor friends who helped us to identify experts, reviewed our questions, and generally pointed us in the right direction: Dr. Joshua Beckman, Dr. Ken Feuerstein, Dr. Mona Gabbay, Dr. Claudia Gold, Dr. Dawn Hershman, Dr. David Hodges, Dr. Jill Leavens-Maurer, Dr. Danny Pine, Dr. Beth Printz, Dr. Carlos Salama, and Dr. Robyn Spirer.

And our deepest thanks to Dr. Mathew Maurer, who helped us to compose many of the questions and reviewed the manuscript for medical accuracy.

After all the doctors were finished reviewing the book, Jeff Kramer, Susan Chong, and Carol Ryan looked at it from a parent's perspective.

Sheri Berger's Web site was the first place we went when we were considering writing this book, and it continued to be one of our most valuable resources.

Rashida and Raghu Mendu of The Heart of a Child Foundation gave tremendous support for this project. We should all thank them for their tireless efforts on behalf of CHD. We hope to see branches of this foundation grow in every town, and more people getting together to raise money for CHD research and relief.

Our thanks also go to our editors, Betsy Rapoport and Stephanie Higgs, as well as to Beth Campbell for her early guidance and to Deborah Schwarz-McGregor at New York Presbyterian Hospital for leading us to our wonderful agent, Robin Dellabough. Thanks, of course, to those people who helped us make the "deal": Art Steinhauer, Paul Thaler, and Noel Silverman. And we very much appreciate the work of our medical illustrator, Rick Gersony, and our friend and photographer, Patty Lipkin.

On a personal note, we want to thank Dr. Emily Jackness, Dr. Jan Quagebour, Dr. Carlyn Opedisano, Dr. Barbara Strassberg, and Dr. Martin Rodriguez-Ema and everyone at Columbia/Babies' Hospital for taking such good care of Lissie and Dr. Michael Meyers, Dr. William Gay, Angela Israel, Dr. Ross Ungerleider, Dr. Martin O'Laughlin, the staff at Duke Hospital, and Dr. James Huhta for taking such wonderful care of Max.

We could not have gotten through any of this without our parents, Ellie and Joel Freid and Stan and Lorraine Berger. Besides sending us to Duke, where we met, they supported us through the kids' surgeries and generally guided us through parenthood over the past seven years. Thanks, too, to all of the Freids, Kramers, Bergers, and Maurers for their encouragement as we wrote this book. And thanks to Jeff, Max, Ethan, Mat, Lissie, Josh, and Eric for letting us sneak away to write and talk and talk and write.

And most of all, our thanks go to Karin Newman Krueger, who had the presence of mind upon hearing about Max's heart defect to say, "Hey,

I think that sounds like what Shari's daughter has. Maybe you two should talk to each other." Without these words we'd have missed each other's support through all of the difficulties that accompany having a child with CHD, and we would never have created this book. Thanks, Karin.

CONTENTS

CONTRIBUTING EXPERTS

Betsy Adler, M.S.N., R.N., C.P.N.P.
Pediatric Nurse Practitioner, Division of Cardiothoracic Surgery
Children's Hospital Medical Center
Cincinnati, Ohio

D. Woodrow Benson, M.D., Ph.D.
Director, Cardiovascular Genetics
Children's Hospital Medical Center
University of Cincinnati
Cincinnati, Ohio

Jonas Ian Bromberg, Psy.D.
Clinical Health Psychologist
Harvard Medical School
Children's Hospital
Boston, Massachusetts

Ruth L. Collins-Nakai, M.D., M.B.A.
President, Canadian Cardiovascular Society
Pediatric Cardiologist
Health Care Consultant
University of Alberta
Edmonton, Alberta, Canada

Amy R. DeFelice, M.D.
Assistant Professor of Clinical Pediatrics
Director of Children's Hospital of New York Nutritional Support Service
Columbia University/New York Presbyterian Hospital
New York, New York

Michael D. Freed, M.D.
Senior Associate in Cardiology, Children's Hospital
Associate Professor of Pediatrics, Harvard Medical School
Boston, Massachusetts

Arthur Garson, Jr., M.D., M.P.H.
Professor of Pediatrics (Cardiology)
Senior Vice President and Dean for Academic Operations

Baylor College of Medicine
Houston, Texas

William Gay, M.D.
Director, Pediatric Specialty Clinic
Roanoke, Virginia

Deborah Gersony, M.D.
Clinical Instructor of Medicine
Columbia University/New York Presbyterian Hospital
New York, New York

Welton M. Gersony, M.D.
Alexander S. Nadas Professor of Pediatrics
Columbia University College of Physicians and Surgeons
Director, Pediatric Cardiovascular Center
Children's Hospital of New York
New York Presbyterian Hospital
New York, New York

Thomas P. Graham, Jr., M.D.
Ann and Monroe Carell Professor of Pediatrics
Director, Division of Pediatric Cardiology
Vanderbilt University Medical Center
Nashville, Tennessee

Kathleen Grima, M.D.
Medical Director
New York Blood Center
New York, New York

James C. Huhta, M.D.
Clinical Professor of Pediatrics
University of South Florida School of Medicine
Tampa, Florida

Emily Jackness, M.D.
Assistant Clinical Professor of Pediatrics
Columbia University College of Physicians and Surgeons
New York, New York

Wahida Karmally, M.S., R.D., C.D.E.
Associate Research Scientist
Director of Nutrition
The Irving Center for Clinical Research
Columbia University
New York, New York

Charles S. Kleinman, M.D.
Adjunct Professor of Pediatrics, Diagnostic Imaging, and Obstetrics and Gynecology

Nemours-Cardiac Center at the Arnold Palmer Hospital for Children and Women
Orlando, Florida
Courteous Clinical Professor of Pediatrics
The University of Florida College of Medicine
Gainesville, Florida

Hillel Laks, M.D.
Professor and Chief, Cardiothoracic Surgery
UCLA School of Medicine
Director, Heart/Heart-Lung Transplant Programs
Director, Alternative Heart Transplant Program
Director, Pediatric and Adult Heart Surgery Programs
UCLA Medical Center
Los Angeles, California

Michael J. Landzberg, M.D.
Director, Boston Adult Congenital Heart (BACH) Service
Brigham and Women's Hospital/Children's Hospital
Harvard Medical School
Boston, Massachusetts
  with special appreciation to
  Susan M. Fernandes, PA-C, Caitlyn O'Brien, PA-C, and Dorothy D. Pearson, PA-C

Ranae L. Larsen, M.D.
Associate Professor of Pediatrics
Loma Linda University Children's Hospital
Loma Linda University School of Medicine
Loma Linda, California

Larry A. Latson, M.D.
Professor and Chairman of Pediatric Cardiology
Medical Director of Center for Pediatric and Congenital Heart Diseases
The Cleveland Clinic Foundation and Ohio State University
Cleveland, Ohio

Peter B. Manning, M.D.
Director, Department of Cardiothoracic Surgery
Children's Hospital Medical Center
Cincinnati, Ohio

Mathew Maurer, M.D.
Assistant Professor of Medicine
Columbia University College of Physicians and Surgeons
New York Presbyterian Hospital
New York, New York

Martin O'Laughlin, M.D.
Associate Professor, Pediatric Cardiology
Duke University Pediatric Cardiovascular Program

Director, Pediatric Cardiac Catheterization Laboratory
Durham, North Carolina

Beth F. Printz, M.D., Ph.D.
Irving Assistant Professor of Pediatrics
Columbia University College of Physicians and Surgeons
New York, New York

Marlon S. Rosenbaum, M.D.
Director, Adult Congenital Heart Disease
Assistant Professor of Clinical Medicine and Clinical Pediatrics
Columbia University College of Physicians and Surgeons
New York Presbyterian Hospital
New York, New York

Amnon Rosenthal, M.D.
Professor of Pediatrics
Michigan Congenital Heart Center
C.S. Mott Children's Hospital
Ann Arbor, Michigan

Kenneth O. Schowengerdt, Jr., M.D.
Associate Professor of Pediatrics
Medical Director, Pediatric Heart Transplant Service
University of Florida College of Medicine and Shands Transplant Center
Gainesville, Florida

Dennis Sklenar, C.S.W.
Senior Pediatric Social Worker
NYU Hospitals Center
New York, New York

Jonathan A. Slater, M.D.
Associate Clinical Professor of Psychiatry (in Pediatrics)
Director, Pediatric Psychiatry Consultation-Liaison Service
Child Psychiatrist, Pediatric Cardiac Transplant Service
Children's Hospital of New York
New York, New York

Ross Ungerleider, M.D.
Professor and Chief, Pediatric Cardiac Surgery
Doernbecher Children's Hospital
Oregon Health Sciences University
Portland, Oregon

Gil Wernovsky, M.D.
Director, Cardiac Intensive Care Unit
Children's Hospital of Philadelphia
Associate Professor of Pediatrics
University of Pennsylvania School of Medicine
Philadelphia, Pennsylvania

Lisa Wispé, M.S.N., R.N., C.P.N.P.
Pediatric Nurse Practitioner, Division of Cardiothoracic Surgery
Children's Hospital Medical Center
Cincinnati, Ohio

Howard Alan Zucker, M.D., J. D.
Associate Professor of Clinical Pediatrics and Clinical Anesthesiology
Columbia University College of Physicians and Surgeons
Associate Attending, Pediatric Cardiology, Critical Care, and Anesthesiology
New York Presbyterian Hospital

FOREWORD

∞

WHEN OUR DAUGHTER, Sophia, was diagnosed with a heart defect, we were overwhelmed. Our baby girl would require open-heart surgery to repair her VSD—a very frightening thought. In our case, we put our trust in her doctors, and from both Sophia's cardiologist, Dr. David Ferry, and her surgeon, Dr. Hillel Laks, we received sufficient information to make intelligent decisions about her care. However, there were times when we had questions. It would have been helpful if a reference book had been available to allay our fears and concerns.

Together, Gerri Freid Kramer and Shari Maurer have written a wonderful book that encompasses many of the issues you will face in the upcoming months and for the rest of your child's life. They have tried to anticipate the questions you will have and provide information you will need to approach your child's health as fully informed as possible.

As we became involved in the congenital heart defect (CHD) community, we learned that there is a broad range of congenital heart defects. This book speaks to all of us, whatever the type and severity of our child's heart defect.

We found it reassuring to read the comments made by other parents. The doctors can give you facts, but those who have been through it personally have much to add to our understanding of life with CHD. The book begins with diagnosis and continues through hospital visits, surgery, and when your grown child starts planning his or her own family. For even after a complete repair, CHD never completely vanishes from your child's life—or yours.

While your doctor is the best source for specific information about your child's condition, use this book as a resource and a friend. Depend on it for support and guidance as your child grows.

Sylvester Stallone and Jennifer Flavin-Stallone

THE PARENT'S GUIDE TO

CHILDREN'S CONGENITAL HEART DEFECTS

INTRODUCTION

∽

WHEN SOMEONE HELD a stethoscope up to each of our tiny newborns' miraculously beating chests and told us there was a problem, a certain amount of innocence and trust was shattered and forever lost. For both of us, it was as if the planets suddenly went out of alignment.

We had met and socialized in college years before, but we didn't keep in touch or send each other birth announcements after we left. Years later, thanks to a mutual friend, we reconnected. We weren't in the same physical community any longer. Unfortunately we were part of a new community, this one made up of parents all over the world who had a child with a congenital heart defect.

Everyone who enters parenthood is forced to suddenly "grow up," but learning your child has a *defect*—what a terrible word—adds an especially heavy measure of responsibility. It's frightening and overwhelming but may be ultimately strengthening.

Not knowing what lay ahead and finding no books about CHD were particularly challenging for us. Technical articles and medical textbooks didn't speak to us. Thankfully, we had each other to call, and some extremely kind, competent physicians.

After both Lissie and Max had surgery, we continued to keep in touch. As we've found, a "repair" doesn't really give you a ticket out of the CHD community. Concerns persist, be they warranted or completely silly, and it's reassuring to be able to talk to someone about them.

Six years later, one thing we can say is thank goodness for E-mail. We can connect at any time of the day or night, and help each other while carrying on with "normal" life. After all, Lissie and Max's lives—and ours with them—are as ordinary and extraordinary as we like them to be.

Somewhere in our correspondence, the idea for this book was born.

We decided to write this book because there was nothing like it when our children were diagnosed with CHD. Along the way, we have discovered a huge CHD community out there, linked together through support groups, friendships like ours, and the Internet. There is a lot more information exchanged among many more parents now than when we began. Yet, the very people who are most involved in the CHD community, who seem to know everything there is to know, are the ones who know just how much this book is needed. Indeed, more than once during the course of compiling and writing it, we have turned to the manuscript for advice with regard to our own children.

Remember that "CHD" encompasses a large and diverse set of physical abnormalities of the heart. Some children with CHD never have surgery, while others need transplants to survive. Some need constant medical attention, others just yearly observation.

We realized from the beginning that CHD is a very broad topic and that it would be difficult to speak to everyone in one book. Yet we've found that from the most common to the most severe defects, we can all learn from each other and all benefit from the support of the CHD community. Along the way, we've had to make decisions about what content would be most beneficial to most readers. As a result, those parents grappling with severe CHD may not find all the answers here. For those parents dealing with less severe CHD, please realize that some of the content of this book will not apply to you and should not cause additional worry, concern, or foreboding.

We encourage you to recognize your unique perspective as you go along.

When you read through the parents' comments, be certain to note the defects associated with their children. Some experiences (such as fear of blood draws) are universal, while others (such as developmental delays) are specific to more severe defects and may not affect your child.

None of the parents in these pages speaks as a medical expert, and not all physicians have the same opinions. For our purposes, our experts answered questions in the most collective of terms. In dealing with your child's specific defect, the answers to certain questions may be different.

We quickly learned that while the field of medicine is full of miracles, nothing in medicine is black and white. What might be right 99 percent of the time might be wrong for your child. And what might be accepted practice today might be replaced by a new theory tomorrow. Consider this book a resource, a guide, and an inspiration. Then trust your instincts and talk to your own physicians.

CHAPTER I

THE DIAGNOSIS

Woodrow Benson, M.D., Ph.D.   James C. Huhta, M.D.

Arthur Garson, Jr., M.D., M.P.H.   Charles Kleinman, M.D.

Thomas Graham, M.D.   Mathew Maurer, M.D.

Amnon Rosenthal, M.D.

L ISSIE was five days old when she was diagnosed as having a heart defect. We were in the hospital treating her for jaundice and the pediatrician, noticing a murmur, referred her to a cardiologist to see what might be wrong. Everyone in the room had such somber looks on their faces, I knew it must be serious, but a voice in my head kept saying, "What's the big deal about a murmur—you hear about people living with murmurs their whole lives. Why is everyone so worried?" The cardiologist who came to see us kindly reassured us that Lissie would be fine. I later understood that she meant that *with surgery* she would be fine.

Receiving a diagnosis of CHD can be overwhelming. There are suddenly many tests for your child to endure, new words and information to digest, and, often, you grope for a reason why. I had made several business trips in my first trimester and convinced myself that the airplane travel must have caused Lissie's defect. Or maybe it was the day I spent in a smoke-filled meeting room in Holland in my seventh week. Or the grape Kool-Aid I drank for the first three months because it was the only thing my nausea could tolerate. (The answer is probably none of these things, but that doesn't stop me from wondering.)

In this chapter we talk about the CHD diagnosis, tests that your child will encounter, possible causes of CHD, and problems you may see in your child's development.

Shari

In the Womb

When is a baby's heart formed?

Dr. Huhta: The baby's heart has formed its chamber and shape by eight to nine weeks of gestation, often before you knew you were pregnant.

I had a sonogram when I was pregnant but no one noticed that my baby had a heart defect until she was born. Why is that?

Dr. Huhta: Most heart defects don't interfere with the early functioning of the heart, which is to pump blood to the body and the placenta. Only after birth, when the lungs are expanded and fully functional, does the problem become obvious. There is a muscular tube called the ductus arteriosus connecting the aorta (main blood vessel to the body) and the pulmonary artery (vessel to the lungs) that stays open before birth. After birth, the ductus closes spontaneously, and this event can lead to blood flow problems in babies with congenital defects.

"I had thirteen sonograms when I was pregnant and they had no idea Joseph had a problem until after he was born. We were absolutely shocked."
—*Katina Doonan, mom to Joseph* (*transposition of the great vessels*)

Didn't my baby's defect affect him when he was in utero?

Dr. Huhta: As long as the heart muscle is pumping normally the valves aren't leaking, and the vessels to and from the lungs and body aren't blocked, then most congenital heart disease is "passive" in utero (before birth). Again, the structure of the heart can be very abnormal, but the function is preserved to maintain normal growth and development, including normal flow to the brain.

My obstetrician said that my baby may have a problem with her heart and recommended a fetal echocardiogram. What is this? Can it hurt the baby or me? What will it be able to tell us?

Dr. Huhta: A fetal echocardiogram is a test using sound waves (ultrasound) to study the structure of your baby's heart before birth. Although your obstetrician may obtain a limited view of your baby's heart during a routine pregnancy ultrasound, a fetal echocardiogram is a very detailed evaluation of your baby's heart by a specialist in fetal echocardiography. There are no known risks to the mother or the fetus. Information is obtained about the details of the structure of the heart (how the valves and chambers are formed) and about the function of the heart as a pump.

The detection of a heart defect increases the risk of finding other malformations in the child. A detailed ultrasound of the rest of the fetus is necessary, and amniocentesis to test the chromosomes may be recommended. If a serious or even life-threatening heart abnormality is identified that will have a significant impact on the future of the child, you'll want to discuss this with your doctor. Currently only cardiac rhythm disturbances are routinely treated in utero, but in the future a number of structural cardiac defects may be repaired before birth.

If a heart defect is found in utero, what can be done about it?
Dr. Huhta: In many cases of CHD diagnosed prenatally, it is safest to deliver the pregnancy at, or near, the medical center at which postnatal treatment will take place, especially if surgery will be required soon after birth.

"Being diagnosed in utero, I had twenty weeks to think positive and negative thoughts. There are pros and cons. You can prepare yourself, find other families who have children with the same problem, educate yourself, other doctors can examine your baby, and you can take more time to make decisions. We were able to change hospitals so I would deliver at the hospital where he would have surgery. But I used to hug my stomach at night and think, 'Please be okay.' "

—Laura Ulaszek, mom to Brian (HLHS)

When do doctors recommend that you terminate a pregnancy?
Dr. Huhta: Most babies with heart defects who have been terminated have had other serious, noncardiac defects, such as brain malformations and genetic problems such as trisomy (extra chromosome). Some heart defects are more serious and only one ventricle (pumping chamber) is present. The key is to get good counseling. The following are suggested:

• A perinatalogist or obstetrician can advise you about the management of the affected pregnancy.

• A pediatric cardiologist is in the best position to give advice about the outlook for your child's heart problem.

• A geneticist can provide information about associated genetic syndromes, if present, and advise about future pregnancies.

• A cardiac surgeon can give you details about any necessary surgical procedures.

• A nurse who is familiar with heart disease in children can provide information about caring for a child with congenital heart disease.

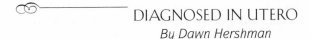

DIAGNOSED IN UTERO
By Dawn Hershman

Getting pregnant wasn't easy for me and my husband. It had taken longer than we thought, and then we had a miscarriage. Finally, several months later, we were pregnant again. My first trimester was a trial. I had multiple episodes of bleeding, and each time I was sure I was having another miscarriage. I had several ultrasounds to make sure the baby was okay. By thirteen weeks the bleeding had stopped, and by twenty weeks I let my guard down.

We went for yet another ultrasound at twenty-two weeks—a test I wanted to cancel, thinking it unnecessary. I remember it very clearly. My husband was late for work. The technician was forty-five minutes late. She started the procedure, I saw the heart beat, and I was reassured. But then I was watching her face and she seemed concerned. She was spending a lot of time looking at the heart. Finally, when I started getting nervous, she explained that there was part of the "pulmonary outflow tract" that she could not see. She immediately sent me for a fetal echocardiogram. Thank God I wasn't alone. I knew something was wrong.

We stood in the waiting room at the pediatric cardiology center. All around us were happy children playing. I couldn't keep the tears from coming. On the walls were beautiful pictures of children and several sentences from each about their lives and their gratitude toward their doctors. Would this be us one day?

I lay on the table usually occupied by small children. I was squeezing my husband's hand so hard it turned blue. I tried to focus on the mobile above my head. When the fetal cardiologist put the probe down and I looked at her face, I felt as if the air had been sucked out of me. "What's wrong?" She was very matter-of-fact. "There is a problem with the heart, but it is very fixable. Let me finish the test and we will talk about it." I didn't hear anything after that.

My head was racing. Being a doctor, all I could think of were bad stories and bad outcomes. My life was not going to be as I planned. What were the long-term repercussions?

We sat in her office as the cardiologist explained that the baby had "transposition of the great arteries." This is a malformation that used to be almost always fatal, but now can be corrected at birth with open-heart surgery. The outcomes are excellent. I could not believe how positive and encouraging she was being. I was numb.

I spent the next couple of days gathering information. I spoke with the department head of pediatric cardiology. He explained the history of this disease. Twenty-five years ago mortality was high; the children had multiple operations. Now, the initial surgery is curative. I could have a vaginal delivery. The baby would be monitored in the NICU [neonatal intensive care unit] after birth. She would have surgery in the first two to three days. She would probably go home a week after the surgery. There would be no monitors at home. There would be a tiny scar. She would lead a normal, active life.

Our job was to get through the next sixteen to twenty weeks. I didn't want this to take away the joy and excitement of pregnancy, but I was scared. We decided only to tell our close friends and relatives, because we didn't want other people to feel sorry for us, and we tried our best to act as if nothing had changed. We tried not to spend too much time thinking "Why me?"

The best thing we did was have dinner with a friend whose daughter had had corrective surgery for a heart defect. She was three when we met her. Nothing was more reassuring than seeing her running up and down the halls of their apartment building. She seemed to have no ill effects. She was a beautiful, happy, healthy child. They were lucky and so were we.

I visited the NICU when I was eight months pregnant, and found it reassuring to meet the nurses beforehand. I felt confident that we were at the right place.

Everything was planned. I was due in December. We were worried about the holidays and doctors being on vacation, so an induction date was scheduled. Unfortunately, my water broke two weeks early, one Friday night after a routine exam. Fortunately, my obstetrician was in town, and she helped coordinate everything. I delivered on Saturday and the surgeon flew back from Europe on Monday night. Our daughter had her surgery on Tuesday, and an uneventful postop course, and we came home the following Monday.

The first year she had four appointments with her cardiologist. Now we go once a year. It took me a long time to get over the constant feeling that something else was going to happen. Once you realize how vulnerable you are—you realize anything can happen, and in a strange way you stop worrying about it.

Every day we tell ourselves that we are so lucky. Our daughter Noa is living proof.

Symptoms and the Diagnosis

Why are some diagnoses made in utero, others at birth, and still others not until a child is older?

Dr. Garson: Diagnosis of congenital heart disease in utero requires an ultrasound specifically directed at the heart of the fetus. Not all fetuses have such a test. Even if they do, occasionally it's very difficult to see structures inside the heart. Most of the time serious congenital heart disease can be diagnosed. Since there are some channels for blood in the fetus that must stay open, certain defects, such as a small atrial septal defect or patent ductus arteriosus, cannot be diagnosed in utero. Some types of congenital heart disease don't produce characteristic murmurs or symptoms until some time after birth (e.g., ventricular septal defect). Other defects (e.g., atrial septal defect) clearly produce symptoms, and the characteristic murmur may be difficult to appreciate.

"When I was first told about Seth, I was looking at the big picture of several operations, etc. It was overwhelming and I was a basket case. Take one day at a time."

—Shelly Corush, mom to Seth (coarctation of the aortic artery, enlarged pulmonary artery, several ASDs and VSDs, surgical heart block)

What is a heart murmur?

Dr. Garson: A heart murmur is simply a noise that usually takes a stethoscope to hear. Commonly, this noise sounds like water running out of the end of a garden hose. Every time the heart beats, there is a "swoosh" that can be heard. Heart murmurs may be either normal or abnormal. In the normal heart, this is simply the sound of normal blood flow as it is being squeezed out of the heart. Children have thin chests, and it's easier to hear normal heart sounds. At some point in their lives, most children have a heart murmur. Murmurs due to an abnormal heart are *less* common than murmurs due to a normal heart. In this case, the passage of the blood through the heart may be abnormal and make a noise, much like a narrowing in a garden hose would make a noise. Some general pediatricians can determine whether a murmur is normal or not. However, if there is uncertainty, a pediatric cardiologist may be asked to listen to the child's heart. If the pediatric cardiologist is uncertain, further diagnostic tests may be performed.

When my baby was first born and they heard a murmur, the doctors told me it might be nothing and go away. Why do some murmurs go away and others don't? What is an innocent or functional murmur?

Dr. Garson: In the first few days of life, a number of important changes occur in the heart and blood vessels of the normal infant. All of these changes occur because when the baby is inside the mother, it doesn't need to breathe, and therefore there is no need for much blood to go to its lungs. While the baby is still in the mother, the main blood vessel that goes to the lungs, the pulmonary artery, has a blood vessel attached to it that allows the blood to go straight from the main pulmonary artery out into the main blood vessel of the body, the aorta. Since this channel is there, very little blood goes into the branches of the pulmonary arteries. After the baby is born, this extra channel between the pulmonary artery and the aorta, called the ductus arteriosus, closes off. This forces a great deal more blood through the side pulmonary arteries. As the ductus arteriosus closes and more blood goes through small pulmonary arteries, heart murmurs may occur, again much like the kink in the garden hose. Over the first few days and weeks of life, these murmurs disappear as the pulmonary arteries enlarge normally.

In infants with congenital heart disease, these changes may cause the appearance of new murmurs. The most common such case is the hole between the two lower chambers, or the ventricular septal defect which, for the first few days and even weeks of life, until the lungs mature, requires increased force to get blood through the lungs. As the amount of blood going through the hole between the left pumping chamber and the right pumping chamber increases, blood flow to the lungs increases.

I can feel my baby's murmur when I touch her chest. Why is that? Does this mean that the defect is very large?

Dr. Garson: You can't tell how serious a defect is by feeling it through the chest. Think of putting your finger under a faucet. When your finger is tight up under the faucet with very little water coming out but making a big spray, this is similar to feeling a heart murmur through the chest. Both small defects and large defects can sometimes be felt through the chest wall. Some very serious defects have no murmurs at all, and some not-so-serious problems make loud murmurs.

"Lissie's murmur was so loud you could hear it across the room and feel it when she was chest to chest cuddling against you."

—Shari Maurer, mom to Lissie (tetralogy of Fallot)

My doctor first said that my child had one problem, then a few weeks later changed the diagnosis. Why is this?

Dr. Garson: As small infants—and their hearts—are growing, the presence and severity of certain defects may change. Some defects that appear large may close; on the other hand, some blocked valves may get tighter and cause more blockage. Additionally, sometimes an impression is based upon a physical examination with a chest X ray and an electrocardiogram. Later, when an echocardiogram is done, the defect becomes better understood.

When should we get a second opinion?

Dr. Garson: If you are unhappy with the care being provided by any physician, it is best to first discuss your displeasure with that physician. If this cannot be resolved, you should seek another physician's opinion. This isn't really a "second opinion" but rather a change of physician. If you have confidence in your physician and understand what the physician is telling you, a second opinion is rarely needed, unless your insurance company requires it. It's always reasonable to ask your physician if there are alternate approaches to treatment and, if there are, why he or she chooses a particular recommendation. If there appear to be alternate types of treatment and the explanations you have received aren't sufficient, then certainly a second opinion would be in order.

"I recommend getting as much information as you can about your child's condition and contacting other doctors to make sure there aren't other options out there that you're not aware of."

—Sharon Popp, mom to Ben
(pulmonary atresia with VSD, transposition of the aorta)

"What I didn't understand at the outset was the severity of the defect. If you don't like the doctor, go to someone else. This is too important."

—Pat Posada Klapper, mom to Alexandra (VSD)

"We had a meeting with her doctors and let them know that we were to be told everything about Shelby's condition, good or bad. Also, we let them know that nothing was to be done to her until we were told about it (tests, procedures, moving her, etc.). The doctors were very responsive to this, and once that was out of the way, things were much better between the doctors and us. Parents should be very up front with the doctors from the beginning and should also remember that doctors are human beings too and are just doing a job."

—Dan and Candy Miller, parents to Shelby (severe pulmonary stenosis)

What is heart failure?

Dr. Garson: In both children and adults, the term "heart failure" describes a group of symptoms. In infants and children, these symptoms are generally rapid breathing, slow feeding, slow weight gain, and profuse sweating—until the clothes are wet. The most common causes for "heart failure" in children are congenital heart defects, where more blood than normal is allowed to go to the lungs (e.g., ventricular septal defect). In such cases, since there is too much blood in the lungs, the vessels in the lungs become stiff, similar to a water balloon, and it becomes easier for the infant to take a large number of shallow breaths rather than the normal number of deeper breaths. Other congenital heart defects may cause heart failure because there is a decrease in the amount of blood being pumped out of the heart into the body. Nonetheless, the major difference between children and adults is that in children, in the vast majority of cases, the function of the heart muscle (its ability to squeeze blood) is normal. This is not the case in adults where, either due to heart attacks or other reasons, the heart muscle may not contract normally.

What should I look for in my baby that might indicate he is in heart failure?

Dr. Garson: The most common early sign of heart failure is that the baby takes a very long time to feed. Most infants require less than twenty to thirty minutes to finish their bottle or breast-feeding; larger infants take in larger quantities, but still don't usually require more than thirty minutes. A great deal of sweating is another important sign. The vast majority of babies sweat some, but if the baby's clothes are wet from sweating during sleeping, this may be a sign of heart failure. Lack of weight gain also may be a sign of heart failure, but may be due to a number of other causes.

My father had heart failure and he's all swollen. Why isn't my baby swollen?

Dr. Garson: The majority of infants and children in "heart failure" don't have swelling. Perhaps this is because they're lying down most of the time; swelling occurs in adults after they've been sitting or standing for a while.

The doctor says my baby is cyanotic. What does that mean?

Dr. Garson: "Cyanosis" means blueness. There are many different causes for blueness, including problems with the heart or the lungs, or rarely, the blood itself. When cyanosis refers to heart disease, it means that there is a congenital heart defect. The blue blood that comes back from the body and that would normally go to the lungs to pick up oxygen instead goes directly back to the body without picking up any oxygen. Children with cyanosis have been referred to as "blue babies." The amount of blueness depends on how much oxygen-poor blue blood bypasses the lungs and goes out to the body. This may change in a baby from minute to minute or over several months. After parents know what to look for, they are the best observers of the degree of blueness in their baby.

Why does my child's heart condition cause him to have trouble breathing?

Dr. Garson: Actually, most children, even those who have a great deal of blood flow to their lungs due to their congenital heart defect, don't have "trouble breathing." They may breathe rapidly since it's easier for babies with some stiffness in their lung blood vessels to breathe rapidly and shallowly. It's unusual for an infant to have "retractions" (where the skin between the ribs indents every time the infant takes a breath in) or flaring of the nose (where the nostrils get larger every time the baby takes a breath in). These are the true signs of "trouble breathing" and if they occur are important to report to your physician.

Why does an enlarged liver sometimes signal a heart problem?

Dr. Garson: In some of the most common kinds of congenital heart defects such as a hole between the two lower chambers (ventricular septal defect), the hole allows too much blood to go into the right side of the heart and into the lungs. This increase in amount of blood in the lungs causes the right side of the heart (right ventricle and right atrium) to work harder to pump this blood. The veins that drain blood into the heart also may get blood "backing up" in them. Since the liver has many veins that drain very close to the heart, when there is some backup of blood within the heart, the veins and the liver itself will enlarge. The liver works much like an oil dipstick in an automobile. It is more of an indicator than a problem in and of itself. It is very unusual for the liver to be damaged by this backup of blood and, in the majority of cases, the heart functions perfectly well and is able to squeeze out the appropriate amount of blood.

What is tachycardia? Bradycardia? How are they controlled?

Dr. Garson: The rate of the heartbeat is largely controlled by nerves that go to the heart. The heartbeat speeds up in times of need such as fever, anxiety, or exercise; it slows down during rest. There is a normal range of heart rates that varies with age. Infants have faster rates and adults have slower rates.

Tachycardia means an abnormally fast heart rate, and bradycardia means an abnormally slow heart rate. Normally the rate varies smoothly, in the same way as a car accelerator. But sometimes the accelerator gets "stuck." The fast heartbeat may come from the top part of the heart (supraventricular tachycardia) or the bottom part of the heart (ventricular tachycardia). Slow heartbeat, or bradycardia, may be caused by a slowing of the normal pacemaker of the heart sinus node (i.e., sinus bradycardia) or injury to the pathway that connects the top and the bottom parts of the heart (AV block). These conditions are rare and also may occasionally occur after heart surgery.

What is an aneurysm of the ventricular septum? Is it like a brain aneurysm? Will it hurt my child?

Dr. Garson: An aneurysm of the ventricular septum looks like a wind sock at an airport—like an outpouching in a blood vessel. In fact, the aneurysm of the ventricular septum is a good thing and is the way that tissue builds up to close a ventricular septal defect (the hole between the two lower chambers). It's also possible to have an aneurysm of the atrial septum.

Tests

What is an X ray? Will it hurt? Does a child with a heart problem undergo a lot of X rays, and can exposure to the radiation have any long-term effects on my child?

Dr. Graham: A chest X ray is a picture of the heart and lungs taken by using radiation. The radiation penetrates different parts of the body to different degrees and thereby generates a picture of your child's internal organs. Typically your child will need to lie down on a table and remain still for a minute or so [the actual X ray penetrates the body in a second or two, but the technician needs to leave the room to take the picture, which adds a few seconds]. The test certainly doesn't hurt, but occasionally some children need to be restrained so that an adequate picture can be obtained. The radiation associated with an X ray is very small and shouldn't have any long-term effects.

"I will never forget the image of my tiny six-day-old baby in restraints as they X-rayed her. They asked me to leave the room because they didn't allow women of childbearing age in the X-ray room."

—*Shari Maurer, mom to Lissie (tetralogy of Fallot)*

What is an EKG? How does it work? Why is it needed? Does it hurt? Will my child need sedation?

Dr. Graham: An EKG, or electrocardiogram, is a test that records the electrical activity of the heart. By placing tiny little electrodes [i.e., stickers] on various parts of a child's chest, the EKG machine can determine differences in electrical activity from different parts of the heart. Your child will lie on the table, and a doctor or technician will place several small stickers on his chest. These stickers will be attached to wires that connect to the EKG machine. An EKG can give your doctor information about the rhythm of the heart and about any changes in the thickness of the heart muscle caused by the heart condition. It doesn't hurt. The child does have to be still for several moments for the test to work, but most technicians can get the child to sit or lie still for long enough to perform the test without using sedation.

What is a Doppler echocardiogram? How does is it work? Why is it needed? Does it hurt? Will my child need sedation?

Dr. Graham: A Doppler echocardiogram, or "echo," as many people call it, is a special test that uses sound waves and computer processing to record a picture of your heart. It's very similar to the sonogram that you may have had while you were pregnant. It's used to learn about how well the heart pumps; the presence of any defects such as valves that don't open enough or are too leaky; and the size, shape, and thickness of the heart chambers. Your child will need to lie on the table, and a jellylike substance will be spread on his or her chest and tummy. The jelly improves the conduction of the sound waves from the ultrasound, giving a clearer picture. The doctor or technician then uses a small probe, which he or she rubs on the jelly. This doesn't hurt; it may just feel a little cold. Your child must lie still for the entire test, which generally takes a half hour to forty-five minutes. Many centers use videos and other forms of distraction (see "Tips for Echos and EKGs"), but in rare situations they will use sedation to make a child groggy and more receptive to the test.

TIPS FOR ECHOS AND EKGS

"Use bubbles, suckers, and their favorite video or TV show. Some people even practice echos at home with an old computer mouse and some Vaseline."

—Susie DeLoach, mom to Joey (HLHS)

"When he was an infant, I would try to make the appointments as close to feeding time as possible and give him a bottle."
—Anne Linne, mom to Kevin (transposition of the great vessels)

"*I* try to be calm."
—Kathy Grampovnik, mom to Beth (aortic stenosis, subvalvular aortic stenosis, and surgical heart block with a pacemaker)

"As a young baby, when Alex was inconsolable during echos, the technicians let me cradle him in my arms or on my lap. That usually helped because it reassured him that as long as he had his mom or dad, then everything was okay, no matter what weird things they were doing on his chest."
—Sara Daniel, mom to Alex (tricuspid atresia, ASD, VSD)

"For echos I have gotten on the table and let her lie back on me."
—Roberta Love, mom to Allison (ventricular inversion, double outlet left ventricle, rudimentary right ventricle, transposition of the great arteries, and VSD)

"When my son was an infant, I actually nursed him during an echo. It was awkward and a little embarrassing, but it kept us from having to sedate him. Now that he's five, diversions like a video are wonderful for helping him to relax and realize that the test doesn't hurt. But he does think that unsticking the electrodes hurts. Finally, I asked the technician if there's a better way and she suggested putting some lotion on Max's chest beforehand (as long as he promised to be very still during the tests) and using an adhesive remover called Uni-Solve to help get the electrodes off."
—Gerri Freid Kramer, mom to Max (tetralogy of Fallot)

"We count for short procedures. During echos we watch videos and blow bubbles."
—Laura Murphy, mom to Amanda (hypertrophic cardiomyopathy and Noonan's syndrome)

"Take a blanket to cover your child during the echocardiogram as they have to be undressed."
—Susan Wirth, nurse and mom to Julia (interrupted aortic arch, VSD, ASD)

"I have talked to Andrew about what to expect in simple terms (for instance during an echo). Even though he's only two, he can understand that someone is going to be touching his chest (or "tummy") and that he will see his heart on TV. I think it helps him to know what's going on and not be surprised."

—*Alisa Spaulding, mom to Andrew (pulmonary atresia)*

My doctor talks about pressures and gradients. What are they, and what do they mean?

Dr. Graham: Pressure is the amount of force the heart generates when it squeezes. The heart should pump the blood by generating enough pressure to force the blood toward the body. When there are heart defects, such as holes (VSD or ASD) or leaky/closed valves, the heart may need to generate more pressure than is normal to continue to do its job. Thus, the pressures measured in the different chambers of the heart give your child's doctor important information regarding how any defect is affecting how hard the heart has to work to perform its job. Pressures can be measured directly by placing a catheter, a long, thin tube (i.e., invasively) in the different chambers of the heart or can be estimated from certain measurements obtained during an echocardiogram.

The gradient is a measurement of the difference in pressure between two parts of the heart. It reflects the severity of the abnormalities of blood vessels and valves. With a VSD (hole in the heart), the gradient goes up as the hole gets smaller, so the bigger the number, the better. With stenosis (narrowing), the gradient increases as the stenosis gets worse, so in that case you want a smaller number.

What is a flow ratio?

Dr. Graham: A flow ratio is the ratio between blood flow to the lungs and to the rest of the body. The normal ratio is 1.0. When there is a defect between the two sides of the heart, there can be flow ratios of 2/1 or 3/1 or higher, indicating that twice or three times as much blood is going to the lungs as to the rest of the body.

What is a cardiac MRI? How does it work? Why is it needed? Does it hurt? Will my child need sedation?

Dr. Graham: A cardiac MRI, or cardiac magnetic resonance imaging, is a series of pictures of the heart and blood vessels made with a large magnet and computer processing. It provides information about anatomy and function of the heart and blood vessels. Your child will need to lie on a table, possibly inside what looks like a tunnel, for usually forty-five minutes. (Newer machines may be called "open" and are not claustrophobic.)

The magnet may make a loud banging noise like a jackhammer as the pictures are being taken. While it doesn't hurt, it may be difficult if your child is claustrophobic. The patient needs to be very still, so it may be easier if your child is sedated.

"Eddie gets an MRI once a year. He's sedated for it—more for the claustrophobia—it doesn't hurt."

—*Robin Yankow, mom to Eddie (aortic stenosis, enlarged aortic root)*

What is a Holter monitor? How does it work? How long does he need to wear it? Does my child need to stay overnight in the hospital while he's wearing it?

Dr. Graham: A Holter monitor is a recording of all the heartbeats for an extended period—usually for twenty-four or forty-eight hours. It provides information on the rate of and rhythm of the heart. The Holter records the heart rhythm from usually three electrodes [i.e., stickers], which are placed on the chest. The electrodes are then attached with wires to a tape recorder that looks like a Sony Walkman. The "Walkman" can be attached to your child's pants or belt for the day. It's important to keep the electrodes well attached so that your child's heart rhythm can be well monitored. It can be worn outside of the hospital and during normal activities.

"At age four, she had to wear a Holter monitor for twenty-four hours. I was concerned about how she would do lugging it with her wherever she went. I needn't have worried! She proudly showed it to everyone she knew and told them it was a tape recorder she could talk into and play back what she had just said."

—*Sheryl Lamb, mom to Heather (double outlet right ventricle,*
hypoplastic right upper chamber, transposition,
subvalvular pulmonary stenosis, bilateral superior vena cava with
interrupted inferior vena cava, common ventricle)

"Max had to wear a Holter monitor when he was a baby. Between nursing, changing clothes often, transporting him in and out of a car seat, and his squirming, the electrodes came off a few times. The technician had told me before I left that if that happened, I could just use Scotch tape to put them back on, so I carried tape everywhere we went, but I was always worried that I didn't get them back on in exactly the right place."

—*Gerri Freid Kramer, mom to Max (tetralogy of Fallot)*

What is angiocardiography? How does it work? Why do they need it? Does it hurt? Will my child need sedation?

Dr. Graham: Angiocardiography is the science of injecting contrast media (dye) into the heart and blood vessels to obtain high-quality X-ray motion pictures. It is performed during cardiac catheterization. Although it's an invasive procedure, it's a good way for your doctor to get information about your child's heart that he can't get from an echo and an EKG. All children who undergo angiocardiography [catherization] require sedation. After cleaning the skin area where the catheter will be inserted, the doctor numbs the skin with some local anesthesia and places a tube into the artery or vein. Doctors then use X-ray images to guide longer tubes [catheters] through the first tube. Once in the correct spot, pressures are recorded and pictures are taken as a dye is injected. During the procedure, your child may feel a warm sensation from the injection of dye, but the procedure itself doesn't hurt. Your child will be sedated and given medication to minimize any pain he might have. (For more about this procedure, see chapter 5.)

What is a tilt table? What is it used for? Will it hurt?

Dr. Graham: If your child is having fainting spells, sometimes referred to as syncope, your cardiologist may recommend a tilt table test to help determine the cause of the fainting. Your child will lie down flat on the table, and the doctor will record the heart rate and rhythm and check his or her blood pressure while your child is lying flat. Then the table will tilt, putting your child in an upright position. While your child is standing, the doctor will continuously record the heart rate and rhythm as well as the blood pressure. The test determines if your child is susceptible to a significant drop in blood pressure that could result in inadequate blood flow to the brain and thus loss of consciousness. While the test doesn't hurt, some patients feel nauseous and light-headed and may pass out during the tilt table test.

What do you learn from blood tests?

Dr. Graham: Blood tests are used for many different reasons. A blood count may be used to try to determine if there is anemia or if there are too many red blood cells being made in response to a cyanotic (blue skin) condition. Your doctor also may draw blood to look for infection, to check kidney function, or to check the electrolytes, which can be altered by a heart condition or by medications. Some medications, such as Coumadin, need monitoring of blood levels and monitoring of the degree of "blood thinning."

"Be up front and honest. Don't say 'It won't hurt' when you know that having blood drawn is gonna hurt. Instead, say 'This is something that has to be done, and it's just going to be a little teeny dinosaur bite and then we will be all done' and again, praise, praise, praise for being brave, etc."

—*Sue Dove, mom to Scott (single ventricle)*

"Having blood work—she will never get used to that . . . she says mean things to me, the phlebotomist, and anyone who helps hold her still."

—*Yolanda Scott, mom to Ondrea (dextrocardia mitral atresia, pulmonary atresia, interrupted IVC, dual permanent pacemaker)*

"We usually give Eddie some EMLA cream so that inserting the IV is less painful. He doesn't like the sensation of the numbness, but we tell him it will help it to be less painful."

—*Robin Yankow, mom to Eddie (aortic stenosis, enlarged aortic root)*

How do you determine which tests to use on my child? Which are the most common diagnostic tests and why?

Dr. Maurer: The tests your child will require are very individualized depending on your child's symptoms, physical examination, and the severity of her condition. Usually, less invasive tests are utilized first to obtain as much information as possible without subjecting your child to undo risk or discomfort. However, certain situations, because of their complexity or severity, require immediate or exact answers that can only be obtained with invasive or somewhat uncomfortable tests. It is important that you understand the risks and benefits of each test. You will be asked to sign an "informed consent" form in which you acknowledge that you understand why a certain test is being performed for your child and what the risks and benefits are. Clearly, being informed and comfortable with the decision to proceed will be conveyed to your child, who is looking for your support and assurance.

FETAL ECHOCARDIOGRAPHY
ITS HISTORY AND USES
By Charles S. Kleinman, M.D.

There have been remarkable accomplishments in the field of prenatal diagnosis and treatment that have been made over the past thirty-five years using fetal echocardiography or ultrasound. Through the use of high-frequency sound waves, at frequencies 100 to 500 times the upper limits of human auditory perception, two- and three-dimensional imaging studies have been used to analyze fetal development.

It should be possible to get an adequate image of the human fetal heart using modern imaging equipment and a transabdominal (on the belly) approach in more than 93 percent of cases, between the sixteenth week of gestation and term. In some cases, in which imaging is compromised because the fetus is too far from the maternal abdominal wall, it may be better to use transvaginal scanning. Using the latter approach, it has been reported that diagnostic studies of fetal cardiac anatomy can be obtained as early as the tenth to twelfth weeks of gestation.

We believe that fetal cardiac examination must be readily available to any woman who is identified to be at high risk for carrying a fetus with congenital heart disease. In recent years, the most important indication for detailed fetal cardiac scanning has been the recognition of an abnormal appearance of the fetal heart on a "nontargeted" ("Level I") or "screening" ultrasound. Such screening studies may result in positive diagnoses in more than 50 percent of referred patients. In contrast, the most *common* single indication for scan in our laboratory remains a previous family history of congenital heart disease, despite the fact that the positive "yield" of these studies varies from only 1 to 2 percent. Although many people wonder if it is cost-effective to do fetal echocardiography studies on the latter group, one should not underestimate the psychological value of a negative cardiac scan to the parents of a fetus thought to be at high risk for congenital heart disease.

When the fetal heart is viewed from a "four-chamber view," it may offer direct visualization of many structural cardiac anomalies (e.g., atrioventricular septal—"canal"—defects; single ventricle; hypoplastic left or right ventricle; mitral or tricuspid atresia), and it should come as no surprise that such profound abnormalities constitute the vast majority of the cardiac anomalies that have been diagnosed worldwide. However, these severe abnormalities do not represent the majority of congenital heart defects. VSD, ASD, and pulmonary stenosis are far more common, but they are very difficult to diagnose through fetal echocardiography and thus often not detected until after birth.

Prenatal cardiac diagnosis can have an important impact on the management of pregnancy, delivery, and the neonatal period. Such information may influence decisions concerning when, where, and how delivery should take place. Most importantly, such information has had important implications concerning parental education and counseling with regard to the crucial issues of informed consent. For the first time, parents faced with life-altering decisions may have the time and information to enable them to formulate decisions after they've had an opportunity to resolve the fear, disbelief, and anger that invariably complicate the initial presentation of tragic information. Clearly, the "traditional" experience of requesting "informed consent" from a physically and mentally exhausted patient within minutes of diagnosis—often in a situation in which the child has been transferred to a cardiac center at a distance from the hospital where delivery has taken place, with consent from a father who may be miles from the mother or alternatively, obtained over the telephone from a distraught, confused, frightened mother who may be recovering from anesthesia or receiving narcotic analgesia—can be avoided.

While prenatal diagnosis may allow parents to decide that the most appropriate course of action for their family is termination of the pregnancy, we have found that this option is rarely pursued when one is dealing with an isolated cardiac abnormality in an otherwise normal fetus. While each family makes decisions in its own unique fashion, the decision regarding termination or continuation of pregnancy often hinges upon information concerning surgical outcomes, and short-, mid-, and long-term functional outcomes for these children. The decision to terminate has been almost exclusively made by parents whose fetus has a form of congenital heart disease that is not amenable to repair into a two-ventricular system. With the excellent short- and midterm outcomes for children with one ventricle that can be managed by Fontan operation or even cardiac transplantation, the decision to terminate pregnancy has become less common. The factors that enter consideration for parents are highly personal and difficult to predict.

As our experience with prenatal diagnosis has expanded, we have been pleased to find that a prenatal diagnosis of complex congenital heart disease increases the baby's chances for survival. This has been most dramatic among newborns with heart malformations that allow repair into two-ventricle pumping systems. While we have just begun a long-term study to prove that prenatal diagnosis provides a neuro-developmental advantage to our patients, we are optimistic that such advantage will be found.

We have witnessed the evolution of the field of "fetal cardiology."

This has developed as an extension of perinatal medicine, neonatology, and pediatric cardiology. The application of ultrasound imaging to establish prenatal cardiac diagnosis may provide parents and physicians with information that is critical for informed management plans that may enhance survival, quality of life, and social adaptation for these infants and families.

Causes of CHD

Is it possible to find out what caused my baby's heart defect?

Dr. Benson: Yes, in many cases. The number of cases of congenital heart defects for which a cause can be identified is increasing at a rapid rate. Ten years ago we recognized a cause in only a small portion of cases. In 1999 we recognized more cytogenetic (chromosome studies) causes and identified a molecular genetic cause (gene mutation) in some cases. The genetic basis of CHD is being recognized with increasing frequency, as exemplified by an increasing number of entries in Online Mendelian Inheritance in Man (OMIM). OMIM is a catalog of human genes and genetic disorders authored and edited by Dr. Victor A. McKusick and his colleagues at Johns Hopkins University, and found on the Web at www3.ncbi.nlm.nih.gov/omim/.

What exposures or activities during pregnancy do most medical experts believe are contributing factors to CHD?

Dr. Benson: Very little is known about specific activities or exposures ("risk factors") for CHD. We do know that some types of maternal illness can affect the developing cardiovascular system of the fetus. For example, infants of mothers with lupus erythematosus, diabetes mellitus, or rubella (German or three-day measles) are known to have increased risk of specific types of cardiovascular problems. In addition, certain medications taken by the mother may affect the fetal cardiovascular system, most notably vitamin A derivatives (used to treat acne). Excessive alcohol use also can affect cardiovascular development in utero.

The March of Dimes Web site (www.modimes.org) has some general guidelines for a maximally healthy pregnancy.

Are there steps that can be taken to prevent CHD?

Dr. Benson: At the present time, we don't know of any. We know that pregnant women who drink alcohol increase the risk of CHD and other birth defects, but we don't know how to reduce risk.

Are some defects genetic? Which ones? What are some of the genetic factors involved in CHD?

Dr. Benson: The simple answer to the first question is "yes" and the answer to the second question is "all of them."

The terms "genetic," "familial," and "inherited" are considered synonyms in dictionaries, but their meanings vary with context. When we use the term "genetic," we mean "relating to the gene or chromosome." Because a genetic or chromosomal abnormality or deletion may occur spontaneously in a baby and have nothing to do with the genes of anyone else in your family, a genetic factor is not always inherited. However, if a genetic factor is also present in other family members, then it is considered inherited. For example, Down syndrome is a genetic condition (trisomy of chromosome 21), but it is rarely inherited or familial. As a second example, a deletion of chromosome 22q11, which is associated with a variety of CHD and may include DiGeorge syndrome, is genetic. Studies have shown that in 15 to 20 percent of cases, the child inherits the deletion from one parent. However, this means that in 80-85 percent of cases, the chromosome 22q11 deletion is sporadic (not inherited), as neither parent has a deletion.

Genetic information is transmitted from parents to their children through genes contained in nuclear chromosomes (autosomes 1–22 and sex chromosomes X and Y) as well as on a single mitochondrial chromosome. In the field of human molecular genetics, genetic refers to DNA (deoxyribonucleic acid), which is the material that makes up chromosomes. The genome (the whole set of genetic material) of humans is made up of 3 billion nucleotides; nucleotides are the building blocks of DNA, and specific arrangements of nucleotides make genes. CHD may occur when there is mutation in the DNA that makes up the chromosomes. Mutations may occur in a number of forms, including duplication or deletion of an entire chromosome, deletion of a segment of a chromosome, or substitution of a single nucleotide.

Some genetic causes or risks of CHD occur on a sporadic basis and some occur on a familial basis. For example, infants with Down syndrome have a high risk of CHD, and the genetic cause usually is sporadic. On the other hand, children with a chromosome 22q11 deletion also have a high risk of CHD. This genetic cause of CHD is sporadic in 80 to 85 percent of cases, but 15 to 20 percent of the time the deletion has a familial basis.

Familial causes of cardiovascular defects can be classified by their patterns of inheritance as autosomal dominant, autosomal recessive, X-linked, or matrilinear (see figure 1). For the cardiologist, recognizing the mode of inheritance can identify individuals at risk of developing these disorders. For the molecular geneticist, patterns of transmission can direct strategies for identification of the responsible gene.

Different modes of inheritance are illustrated in figure 1. With *autosomal-dominant disorder*, the offspring of affected individuals have a 50 percent chance of inheriting this condition. Familial supravalvular aortic stenosis, which occurs in male and female family members in each generation, is one example.

With autosomal-recessive inheritance, both parents are unaffected carriers, and approximately 25 percent of their offspring will be affected. Affected siblings without affected ancestors may indicate autosomal-recessive inheritance. CHD, usually a large atrial septal defect or common atrium, is common in Ellis–von Creveld syndrome, which is inherited as an autosomal-recessive trait. Since the incidence of recessive-gene defects in the general population is low, the risk that an affected individual will transmit the disorder to their offspring is small.

CHD that occurs only in male family members suggests an *X-linked disorder*, a disorder linked to the X-six chromosome. The male offspring of affected men will not be affected, but the offspring of unaffected women are at risk. A form of visceral heterotaxy has been shown to be inherited in an X-linked manner.

With matrilinear inheritance, all of the offspring of affected women but none of the offspring of affected men are at risk of disease. Kearn-Sayres syndrome, which is associated with a high risk of developing atrioventricular block, is inherited in a matrilinear fashion.

The situations shown in figure 1 account for very little of CHD. More often the picture is confused by variable expressivity (diversity of CHD in family members bearing the gene mutation) or reduced penetrance (the absence of a clinical problem in some individuals bearing the gene mutation). These concepts are illustrated in figure 2. The left side of figure 2 represents the extended family of a young girl (blackened round symbol) who has CHD—let's say an atrial septal defect (ASD). When her parents are asked about family history, no one else is known to have ASD. The family history appears to be negative. This is often the case for CHD. However, at the next visit, the parents provide some additional information obtained from family members. (This new information is represented by the revised history on the right side of figure 2.) At age fifty years, the patient's grandfather (gray box) had surgery for replacement of a heart valve, and the patient's aunt (gray circle) was said to have had a "hole in the heart" that closed spontaneously during childhood. One genetic implication of this

Figure 1. Models of Mendelian inheritance.

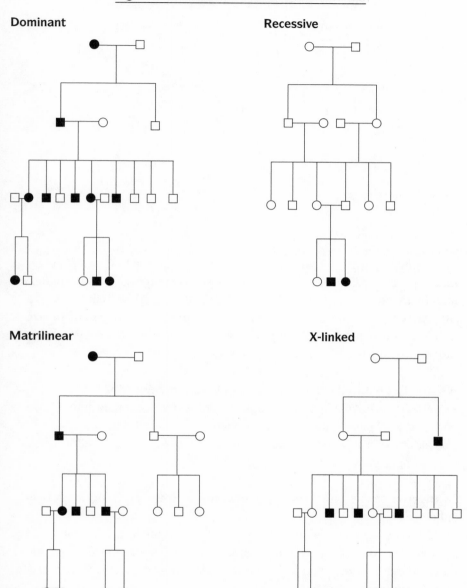

new information is that in this family CHD is inherited in an autosomal-dominant manner. Individuals who inherit the disease gene have different types of CHD (variable expressivity), and some individuals appear to have none at all (reduced penetrance). Molecular genetic studies have identified a number of examples of this scenario.

Figure 2: Pedigrees with two clinical scenarios.

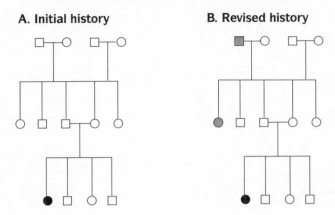

A. Initial history   B. Revised history

Ultimately, with the identification of disease genes that result in cardiac defects, we'll be able to make more precise diagnoses, better understand why and how CHD affects people, identify who's at risk for it, and offer better treatment to those who have it. Moreover, if we can recognize individuals who have inherited gene defects but have not developed a heart defect, we may be able to delay the onset of symptoms.

No one in my family has CHD. Could it still be genetic?

Dr. Benson: Yes. Sporadic mutation, autosomal-dominant inheritance with reduced penetrance, and autosomal-recessive inheritance would fit this situation. These are classic situations where a genetic condition may not be apparent from family history.

Is there a test to determine whether—or how—my baby's CHD is inherited?

Dr. Benson: There is no single test available to answer this question. A combination of careful, detailed family history and assessment of the baby's condition may lead to a recommendation to use cytogenetics or a specific mutation analysis.

Should we see a genetic counselor?

Dr. Benson: At present there are no generally accepted guidelines for seeing a genetic counselor. This is a question to discuss with your child's cardiologist.

How can we be sure that genetic information about our family is kept confidential?

Dr. Benson: No national guidelines or regulations prohibiting use of genetic information in a discriminatory manner have been established. However, at least thirty-three states have passed laws that prohibit insurance companies from using genetic information to set premiums or deny insurance coverage.

I've read that a lot of defects are associated with syndromes. What are some of the most common syndromes? Should my child undergo special testing to find out if she has one of these syndromes?

Dr. Benson: A syndrome is a constellation of findings, usually involving many systems. Common syndromes include Down syndrome, Williams's syndrome, Holt-Oram syndrome, Turner's syndrome, and Noonan's syndrome. Usually the syndrome is diagnosed on clinical grounds, and concern about the possibility of a syndrome is one reason to see a clinical geneticist. In many cases a genetic test can be performed that confirms or refutes the impression of a syndrome. By knowing what you're dealing with, you can capitalize on the experience of others and anticipate future problems known to be part of the syndrome. Additionally, you may learn about whether other or future family members have a risk of the same problem.

Are any other structural abnormalities associated with CHD?

Dr. Benson: In most cases, CHD is the only anomaly, but there are exceptions. For example, in Holt-Oram syndrome, the arm is usually malformed.

What is a teratogen?

Dr. Benson: Any environmental agent that produces or increases the likelihood of fetal harm is termed a teratogen. Such agents include microorganisms, substances, or maternal conditions capable of disrupting the fertilized ovum, embryo, or fetus. In most cases the precise way in which environmental exposures cause abnormal development in a fetus is not fully understood. According to the medical specialty of teratology, before an agent can be classified as a teratogen, other causes of fetal harm must be ruled out. Then the agent's cause-and-effect relationship must be carefully identified, defined, and proven. Thus far, only a few agents have met these criteria.

What new studies are under way about the causes of CHD?

Dr. Benson: The field of molecular genetics is making discoveries about the genetic causes of CHD at a very fast pace. These include family studies as well as screening affected individuals for mutations in known genes.

"I took my prenatal vitamins, didn't drink, did everything right—I don't know why this happened. The doctors tell you that it's nothing you did, but you never really believe it."

—*Carole Stoll, mom to Zachary*
(VSD, subaortic stenosis, interrupted aortic arch)

"Every once in a while a little part of me thinks I had something to do with the problem. No matter if friends try to tell me different."

—*Michelle Goenner, mom to Alyssa Mae*
(dextrocardia, heterotaxy asplenic syndrome,
double outlet right ventricle, severe pulmonary stenosis)

"Love your child completely for who he is. Don't dwell on why this happened. Simply move on and throw everything you have into loving your child because you realize that life, any life, is precious and a gift."

—*Sara Daniel, mom to Alex (tricuspid atresia, ASD, VSD)*

Development

Will my child reach his developmental milestones on time?

Dr. Rosenthal: Most children born with heart disease will grow and develop normally. Some variability in reaching milestones is to be expected among children, and significant delay may occur in some children with serious heart disease. Development among infants and children with heart disease depends on the type of heart defect or disease and often on the presence of other associated health problems such as intrauterine growth retardation, prematurity, major anomalies in other body systems, or genetic disorders. Children with congestive heart failure or cyanotic heart problems usually walk and talk one to four months later than other children. Over the past few decades, the outlook for the child with congenital heart disease has greatly improved because surgical repair is performed at an early age. Improvements have been made in operative techniques and anesthesia for children, and there has been considerable development of dedicated postoperative cardiac intensive care units. All these advances should result in improved developmental outcomes for children.

Will my baby develop normally?

Dr. Rosenthal: The great majority of infants and children born with congenital heart problems develop normally. However, some may have motor, perceptual, or intellectual delays. Most of these children have obvious explanations for the developmental delay, which tends to be apparent early in life. Coexisting genetic or other abnormalities in the central nervous system or musculoskeletal system may lead to major or subtle developmental abnormalities. Chronic congestive heart failure or cyanosis in infants may delay weight or height maturation as well as motor or cognitive skills. Providing the child with a stimulating and loving environment while at the same time avoiding being overly protective will maximize your child's developmental potential.

"Alex's gross motor development (sitting up, standing) has been delayed as a result of his CHD. At the advice of our doctors, we went through Child and Family Connections—Early Interventions program in our state (Illinois) and have a physical therapist come to our house once a week to help Alex catch up to other kids his age (free of charge to us, paid for by the state)."

—*Sara Daniel, mom to Alex (tricuspid atresia, ASD, VSD)*

"Joey is delayed in gross motor skills. I knew from about seven months that he wasn't doing what he should be doing. Joey hated being on his belly. After what he had been through we didn't force the issue, didn't want to make him do things he didn't want to do. Big mistake. All of a child's gross motor skills begin from the movements they learn while on the belly. We didn't know this. He started physical therapy at thirteen months. At that time he couldn't even get to sitting from lying down by himself. He started crawling at seventeen months. He walked at twenty-two months, but part of that was due to him having low muscle tone in his ankles. He is still in therapy at two years and we are working on running and jumping. He'll catch up!"

—*Susie DeLoach, mom to Joey (HLHS)*

Will she have any developmental setbacks after surgery?

Dr. Rosenthal: Heart surgery usually enables children to enjoy increased stamina and vigor, better weight gain, enhanced level of activity, and normal developmental milestones. Surgery performed in infancy will often lead to catch-up weight and height. Postoperative improvements depend on the extent and severity of the preoperative problems, genetic factors, coexisting conditions, how successful the operation is, and the persistence of any medical problems. In a very small number of children, a neurologic complication such as a stroke may occur following surgery, and this may subsequently lead to subtle or major developmental problems. Some behavioral or emotional regression may occur subsequent to surgery or hospitalization, particularly in children between the ages of two and four years. Preparing your child, bringing familiar objects to the hospital, and rooming-in help to minimize adverse reactions.

My child's intellectual development seems delayed. What factors specific to CHD affect intellectual development?

Dr. Rosenthal: Impaired intellectual development in a child with heart disease is not necessarily the result of the heart condition. Whatever caused the infant to be born with a heart abnormality may have at the same time led to the development of abnormalities in other systems, including the brain.

That said, a number of factors in infants and children with congenital heart disease may lead to impaired intellectual development. These include chronic hypoxemia (cyanosis), congestive heart failure, associated genetic abnormalities and major noncardiac malformations, low-birth weight (prematurity or intrauterine growth retardation), poor nutrition, or coexisting conditions such as anemia (low red blood cell count) or low level of thyroid hormone.

The effect of low oxygen or cyanosis on development depends on its severity and duration. Prolonged cyanosis may lead to slightly lower IQ, as well as poor perceptual and gross motor function. Congestive heart failure typically results in delayed developmental milestones, and the combination of long-term cyanosis and heart failure can be particularly detrimental. Anemia, or low blood count, may, in individuals with cyanosis, lead to less oxygen being delivered to the brain and thus result in adverse changes. Similarly, the infant with heart failure and diminished blood flow to the head and a low blood count may also be adversely affected. The combination of low blood oxygen, poor blood flow, and anemia will, if persistent, lead to impaired intellectual development or other central nervous system complications. Perceptual motor functions are generally more impaired than cognitive function in a child with heart disease, possibly due to long periods of reduced physical activity or prolonged hospitalization.

What factors specific to open-heart surgery affect intellectual development?

Dr. Rosenthal: Most major heart operations, referred to as open-heart surgery, are performed in infants and children using a heart lung machine (cardiopulmonary bypass) or complete heart stoppage at very low temperature (hypothermic circulatory arrest). There are multiple modifications and combinations depending on the type of heart condition or body size. Prolonged hypothermic circulatory arrest time, particularly when greater than forty-five minutes, may result in decreased intellectual function, whereas long cardiopulmonary bypass or continuous hypothermia bypass at reduced flow rates seems to have fewer effects on the central nervous system. Hypothermic circulatory arrest tends to have a greater effect on performance of nonverbal skills, rather than language skills. The longer the period of arrest, the more likely that neurologic complications will occur.

In addition to cardiopulmonary bypass and circulatory arrest time, other preexisting perioperative or postoperative factors may influence intellectual development. Poor blood flow or insufficient oxygen delivery to the central nervous system may occur at any time among the induction of anesthesia, throughout the surgery, or in the postoperative period. Other postoperative factors that may influence subsequent cognitive skills or adaptive or emotional changes include arrhythmias, blood clots or thromboses, brain swelling, infections, or severe adverse reactions to medications. Visual motor integration deficits are more prevalent in complex congenital heart disease and following multiple operative procedures.

REACTIONS TO THE DIAGNOSIS

"Joey isn't old enough to understand that he has a heart defect. What amazes me is that the little guy has no idea anything is wrong with him. He just plays and whines for juice like any other toddler."

—*Susie DeLoach, mom to Joey (HLHS)*

"When Kevin was born and we found out he had a heart defect, we were scared, shocked, and sad. I thought this helpless little boy, if he lived, would probably be sickly and weak and require a lot of special care. I was willing to give him anything he needed. I just wanted him to come home. Much to my constant amazement, he is a very energetic, busy little boy. He's been on no medication since he came home, and his reports from the cardiologist have been excellent."

—*Anne Linne, mom to Kevin (transposition of the great vessels)*

"Having a chronically ill child certainly makes one consider the fragility of life, even for the very young."

—*Laurie Beard, mom to Trevor (tetralogy of Fallot, Down syndrome)*

"Sometimes her scar will show and someone will ask me what happened. I don't hold back on telling them what she's been through. I'm actually proud to tell them her story."

—*Michelle Goenner, mom to Alyssa Mae*
(dextrocardia, heterotaxy asplenic syndrome,
double outlet right ventricle, severe pulmonary stenosis)

"Don't give up. My son was only 3.8 pounds and 12 days old when he went through his first surgery. He was given a 50 percent chance of survival, and the doctor was morbid about the whole thing. I asked every question I could until I was sure I understood completely about what causes it, what they need to do with each surgery, and how he was going to be afterward as well as complications. I am determined for this not to keep my son down."

—*Dawn Howie, mom to Travis (HLHS)*

"It's funny the different things that you worry about—my husband was worried that he wouldn't be able to wrestle with her."

—*Sheryl Lamb, mom to Heather, (double outlet right ventricle,*
hypoplastic right upper chamber, transposition,
subvalvular pulmonary stenosis, bilateral superior vena cava with
interrupted inferior vena cava, common ventricle)

"Most of all, I enjoy Amanda, and everything she has overcome gives me strength and hope for the next hurdle. And sometimes I forget (briefly) that we have any issues at all."

—*Laura Murphy, mom to Amanda*
(hypertrophic cardiomyopathy and Noonan's syndrome)

"Personally, I have found some wonderful things that have emerged from our challenges—like the ability to appreciate each and every moment with our two children in a way I don't know would be possible without this diagnosis. We learned very early on to live with no regrets."

—*Laurie Strongin, mom to Henry (tetralogy of Fallot)*

"Psyche yourself for the worst and be pleasantly surprised when it's not that bad."

> —*Joanne Baldauf, mom to Kenny (double inlet left ventricle with an outflow chamber and transposition of the great vessels)*

CHAPTER 2
COMMON CONGENITAL HEART DEFECTS

Deborah Gersony, M.D.

OKAY, so now you have a specific diagnosis. Your child's heart defect has a name. When Lissie was diagnosed with tetralogy of Fallot, we wanted to know as much as possible about what lay ahead for her, both in the short and the long term. This chapter will address many of your questions.

We have chosen to define the most common defects. Many children have complex defects, combining two or more of the common ones. As always, each child is different, even children with the same defect, and your doctor is the best source of specific information. Lissie and Max were both born with tetralogy of Fallot. When Max was born, Lissie was seven months old. She had not had her surgery yet. She was not blue and not suffering from any spells. Since she was growing and stable, her doctors were waiting for her to get older and stronger before operating. The first time Gerri and I spoke, it seemed as if the two children had very similar cases of tetralogy and that Max, too, would wait until he was older for his surgery. However, Max's situation became more acute and he wound up having his repair much earlier than the doctors had originally thought. It is important to keep in mind that just because another child has the same defect as yours, the treatments may not be identical.

In this chapter, Dr. Deborah Gersony has provided an overview of each defect. She gives a definition of the defect and then talks about the possible symptoms, the prognosis, and the medical and surgical treatment options. She continues with restrictions, long-term concerns, and future medical advances.

We have also included pictures showing how each defect compares to a normal heart. I know that it greatly helped my understanding of Lissie's heart when her cardiologist drew a picture of a normal heart and then showed me what a heart with tetralogy looked like.

As with the rest of the book, we want this section to be a jumping off point for discussion with your child's doctor.

Shari

NORMAL HEART: EXTERNAL AND INTERNAL

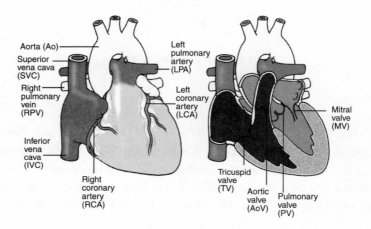

NORMAL HEART: CORONARY ARTERIES AND FOUR-CHAMBER VIEW

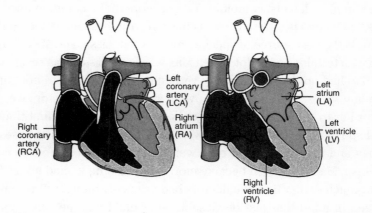

Name of defect: Anomalous origin of the left coronary artery from the pulmonary artery

Definition/anatomy: In this condition, the left coronary artery originates from the pulmonary artery instead of the aorta.

Possible symptoms: Infants cannot complain of chest pain when they exert themselves, so symptoms of this defect are difficult to assess. Affected babies often become irritable, crying and sweating after feeding and

ANOMALOUS ORIGIN OF THE LEFT CORONARY ARTERY FROM THE PULMONARY ARTERY

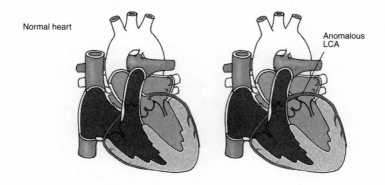

bowel movements. Sometimes the defect results in a heart attack and heart failure with significant leaking from the mitral valve. Occasionally, because small vessels called collaterals grow and supply blood to the left ventricle, symptoms do not develop until later in life. In these cases, the defect is detected after the child complains of chest pain with exercise.

Prognosis: This was once a universally fatal disease, but now the prognosis is quite good. Many studies have shown that even when an infant has a heart attack, the heart muscle recovers very well after surgical correction.

Treatment and surgical options: The treatment of choice in these patients is surgery to reconnect the left coronary artery into the aorta from the pulmonary artery. Mitral regurgitation (leaking) dramatically improves after corrective surgery.

Surgical timing: Generally, the corrective surgery should be performed at the time of diagnosis.

Medications and medical care postsurgery: Medical treatment is indicated in infants with congestive heart failure and abnormal heart rhythms.

Possible restrictions: Once corrective surgery is performed, the child's exercise should be limited only if he or she has significant symptoms.

Long-term concerns: Infants who have had a heart attack may have decreased heart function or leaking of the mitral valve. Such children need to be followed closely, and occasionally medications such as digitalis and diuretics are required.

Medical advances to watch for: New ways to assess the coronary arteries that don't require cardiac catheterization are rapidly developing. These techniques include magnetic resonance imaging (MRI) and ultrafast CT scanning.

ATRIAL SEPTAL DEFECT (ASD)

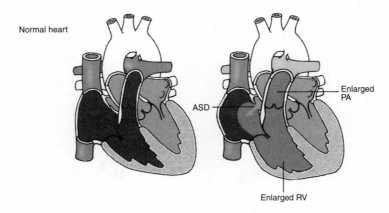

Normal heart

Enlarged PA

ASD

Enlarged RV

Name of defect: Atrial septal defect (ASD)

Definition/anatomy: An ASD is a hole in the wall that divides the top two chambers of the heart (the right and left atrium). The hole can be in different sections of the wall. The most common type of ASD is called a secundum ASD. This type of defect is near the center of the dividing wall. The other types of ASD include: Sinus venosus ASD, high on the wall between the two atria and often associated with *anomalous pulmonary venous drainage* and ostium primum ASD, lower on the wall between the two atria.

Possible symptoms: Children with an ASD usually have no symptoms.

Physical exam: The cardiologist will often hear a murmur and a "fixed splitting" (a short delay between the closing of the aortic valve and the closing of the pulmonic valve) of one of the heart sounds. These findings can be quite subtle. For that reason, doctors occasionally miss the diagnosis of a simple secundum ASD, and the condition may not be identified until adulthood.

Prognosis: Excellent. This is a simple cardiac defect that is easily closed in the operating room or in the cardiac catheterization laboratory.

Treatment and surgical options: The classic treatment of an ASD is surgical closure. In a newer treatment, some ASDs can be closed with a device that can be placed while in the cardiac catheterization laboratory.

Surgical timing: A secundum ASD of any size should be watched for the first one to two years because these defects often get much smaller or even close spontaneously during this period. If the child still has the defect by two to three years of age, it should be closed to prevent progressive heart disease much later in life. Very tiny ASDs generally don't require closure.

Medications and medical care presurgery: None.

Medications and medical care postsurgery: None.

Possible restrictions: None.

Long-term concerns: Occasionally, later in life after closure of an ASD, patients may have a problem with palpitations from abnormal heart rhythms. These rhythms come from the right or left atrium and usually can be treated with medications or therapy in the electrophysiology laboratory.

Medical advances to watch for: The technology that enables a simple secundum ASD to be closed with a device that is placed without surgery may become the treatment of choice in the future.

COARCTATION OF THE AORTA

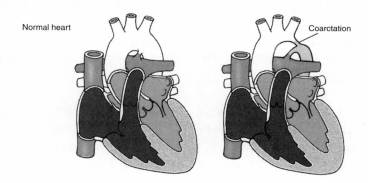

Normal heart

Coarctation

Name of defect: Coarctation of the aorta

Definition/anatomy: Coarctation of the aorta is a localized narrowing of the aorta just after it gives off the vessels to the head, neck, and arms. This cardiac malformation can be associated with other defects, such as bicuspid aortic valve (an abnormality of the valve in which two leaflets are present instead of three), VSD, and mitral valve disease.

Possible symptoms in infants: If the narrowing in the aorta is very tight, infants can have heart failure. Symptoms include rapid breathing and failure to thrive.

Possible symptoms in children: Most children with coarctation of the aorta do not have symptoms.

Physical exam: These children will have higher than normal blood pressures in the arms. The cardiologist or pediatrician may notice that the pulses in the legs are somewhat weak and sluggish compared to the pulses in the arms. Often a heart murmur can be heard.

Prognosis: Favorable. Sometimes children continue to have high blood pressure after surgical or transcatheter correction of the coarctation. High blood pressure must be carefully followed.

Treatment and surgical options: Generally, coarctation of the aorta is corrected surgically. There is a 5 to 10 percent chance that the narrowing will return many years after correction. In this case, dilatation of the narrowing with a balloon or a device called a stent is quite successful in the cardiac catheterization laboratory.

Surgical timing: If the coarctation is severe, then it must be corrected immediately, even in the first few days of life. A routine "adult-type" coarctation (a narrowing that is not critically small) should be corrected in early childhood to prevent persistent high blood pressure.

Medications and medical care presurgery: Medicines such as digitalis may be needed prior to surgical repair to help the heart pump the blood through this tight narrowing.

Medications and medical care postsurgery: Infants and children will need to stay in a special cardiac care unit until they recover from surgery, which varies from child to child. Long-term medical treatment depends on the child's blood pressure after surgery or the presence of associated defects.

Possible restrictions: Heavy weight lifting is generally not recommended for these patients. Otherwise, no significant restrictions are necessary. Antibiotic prophylaxis should be given before dental procedures.

Long-term concerns: In 5 to 10 percent of cases, the coarctation may recur. Therefore, children need yearly examinations, with blood pressure measurements in the arms and legs.

Medical advances to watch for: The technology used for opening up the narrowed area of the aorta is rapidly advancing. In some cases, procedures such as stenting (using a tube to prop open an artery) can be used during catheterization, instead of surgery, for the first correction.

CORONARY ARTERY FISTULAS

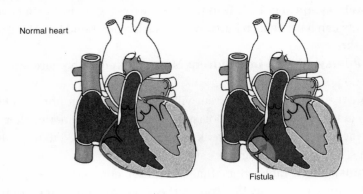

Normal heart

Fistula

Name of defect: Coronary artery fistula

Definition/anatomy: A coronary artery fistula is an abnormal connection between a coronary artery and one of the four cardiac chambers or pulmonary artery. The most common chambers involved are the right ventricle and the right atrium.

Possible symptoms: Most infants and children have no symptoms and are referred to a cardiologist because of a murmur.

Prognosis: The prognosis after successful closure of a coronary artery fistula is excellent. Occasionally a very small communication closes on its own.

Treatment and surgical options: The fistula can be closed either in the cardiac catheterization laboratory with a technique called coil embolization or in the operating room by directly closing the abnormal connection.

Surgical timing: In most cases the abnormal connection is closed even if the patient has no symptoms, because of the risk of future complications such as infective endocarditis (an infection of the heart) or later coronary disease.

Medications and medical care presurgery: Prior to dental procedures, patients will need prophylactic antibiotics.

Medications and medical care postsurgery: None

Possible restrictions: None

Long-term concerns: Patients who have a corrective procedure have an excellent prognosis without long-term adverse events.

Medical advances to watch out for: Improved techniques to close these coronary fistulas in the cardiac catheterization laboratory are under development.

EBSTEIN'S ANOMALY

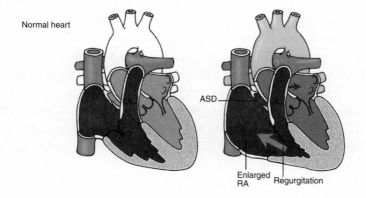

Normal heart

ASD

Enlarged RA   Regurgitation

Name of defect: Ebstein's anomaly of the tricuspid valve

Definition/anatomy: Ebstein's anomaly is a malformation of the right-sided tricuspid valve in which the valve is abnormally low in the right ventricle. This leads to an enlarged right atrium and a "leaky" tricuspid valve. Sometimes blood is pushed through a small hole in the wall between the right and the left atrium, which results in deoxygenated blood going to the body. This shunting can lead to "cyanosis" or a blue discoloration most noticeable on the nails and lips.

Possible symptoms: The symptoms for this form of congenital heart disease vary. If the valve is only mildly abnormal, infants and children may be symptom-free until well into adulthood. Infants may have a cardiac murmur, congestive heart failure (symptoms include difficulty feeding, excessive sweating, and poor growth), and cyanosis (blue discoloration of the fingernails and lips). The symptoms seen in infants may become less apparent within weeks, as the lungs mature. In adulthood, symptoms may be shortness of breath with exertion and fatigue, but are most often related to palpitations (arrhythmia).

Prognosis: The prognosis for this anomaly is variable. Many patients do well for decades. If the defect is very severe, it may not be correctable with surgery. In some cases, patients may need palliative surgery very early in life.

Treatment and surgical options: In patients with symptoms, the tricuspid valve can be repaired with surgery, and any holes in the wall between the left and the right atrium closed.

Some patients may have problems with arrhythmia originating in the area of the abnormal tricuspid valve. This syndrome is called Wolff-Parkinson-White syndrome or "preexcitation" and can be very serious. If this syndrome is detected, it can be cured either in the cardiac electrophysiology laboratory or surgically in the operating room.

Surgical timing: The timing of surgical correction depends on the severity of the malformation and symptoms. Infants with significant cyanosis and heart failure may need early surgery, but the outlook still may be poor. If symptoms are mild, then correction may be carried out later in life. Some patients have no symptoms at all. They should be watched carefully by a cardiologist because they may eventually need surgery.

Medications and medical care postsurgery: Patients need intensive care monitoring after surgery. The typical hospital stay is five to seven days. All patients (both corrected and uncorrected) need prophylactic antibiotics prior to dental work.

Possible restrictions: After correction the patient has no specific restrictions.

Long-term concerns: Arrhythmias are common in these patients. Any complaints of palpitations should be evaluated by an electrophysiologist (a cardiologist who specializes in abnormal heart rhythms).

Medical advances to watch for: Improved methods to treat or prevent cardiac arrhythmias.

ENDOCARDIAL CUSHION DEFECT/AV CANAL DEFECT

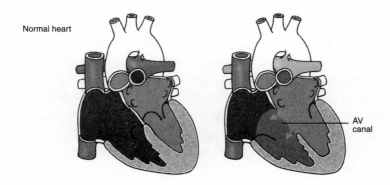

Name of defect: Endocardial cushion defect/AV canal defect

Definition/anatomy: An endocardial cushion defect is a hole in the area where all four chambers meet (left and right atria, and left and right ventricles). This includes the mitral and tricuspid valves. Endocardial cushion defects range from a small opening between the two atria (primum ASD) to a large hole in the center of the heart that causes an opening between the ventricles as well as between the atria. Sometimes the mitral and tricuspid valves become joined into a "common valve," which is insufficient (it leaks). This defect is often associated with congenital syndromes such as Down syndrome.

Prognosis: The prognosis of this congenital defect depends on the extent of the abnormality.

Treatment and surgical options: Ostial primum ASDs are surgically correctable. This "partial av canal" defect is almost always associated with some degree of mitral valve disease. If significant "leaking" is present, the mitral valve may need to be repaired as well. Complete AV canal defects require more intricate surgery, involving patch closure of the atrial and ventricular openings and repair of the mitral and/or tricuspid valves. Occasionally the mitral valve is deformed enough to require replacement.

Surgical timing: Generally, large AV canal defects should be repaired within six months of life, because permanent lung damage can result from prolonged exposure to high blood flow in the pulmonary vessels. If a child has primum ASD and mild mitral valve disease, it is reasonable to wait until just before he or she starts school to undergo repair.

Medication and medical care presurgery: Complete AV canal defects require corrective surgery to eliminate shortness of breath and cyanosis. Patients may require medicines such as digitalis and diuretics prior to the operation.

Medication and medical care postsurgery: All patients need specialized care in an intensive care unit after surgery. Typical hospital stay after a full repair is seven to ten days.

Possible restrictions: After surgical correction, no specific restrictions apply. Patients need prophylactic antibiotics before dental procedures.

Long-term concerns: After a complete repair, many patients will have some leaking of the left-sided mitral valve. Occasionally there is a narrowing below the aortic valve, called subaortic stenosis. These residual defects should be monitored carefully by a pediatric cardiologist. If the surgery for a complete AV canal defect isn't done early enough, the child may develop disease of the arteries in the lungs.

HYPOPLASTIC LEFT HEART SYNDROME

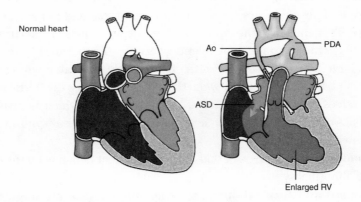

Name of defect: Hypoplastic left heart syndrome

Definition/anatomy: This syndrome includes several cardiac defects that involve underdevelopment of the left side of the heart. These structures primarily include the left ventricle and the aorta. The left-sided valves (aortic and mitral) may be completely closed, meaning all blood must be pumped by the right ventricle alone.

Possible symptoms: Infants usually have heart failure in the first week of life; symptoms include poor feeding, failure to grow, and profuse sweating.

Prognosis: Untreated patients live only for a few days or weeks. After complex staged surgery, many patients do well for many years. However, there are often late manifestations. In some cases, infants or children are treated with cardiac transplant.

Treatment and surgical options: During the first stage of the palliative surgery called the "Norwood procedure," named after the surgeon who developed it, the one existing ventricle is connected to the aorta and the connection to the lungs is closed off. The blood flow to the lungs is then restored by connecting the subclavian artery to the pulmonary artery. During the second stage of the procedure, blood flow is routed to the lungs from the artery to a vein in the chest (Glenn operation). A third stage consists of an operation to direct all venous flow into the lungs (Fontan procedure).

Surgical timing: The first stage of the procedure is carried out within the first few weeks of life. The second stage is usually performed between six and nine months of age. The third stage is usually carried out near three years of age.

Medications and medical care presurgery: Medical therapy does not play a large role prior to surgery.

Medications and medical care postsurgery: Therapy after surgery may include a medicine called digoxin to help the right heart pump strongly in the postoperative period; if the patient has heart failure, a diuretic may be necessary. Anticoagulation medicines such as aspirin or warfarin are prescribed for some patients who have the Fontan procedure.

Possible restrictions: Generally, these children can't exercise as vigorously as other children of the same age, and are advised to avoid contact sports and extreme forms of exertion. They need prophylactic antibiotics before dental procedures.

Long-term concerns: There are several important long-term concerns for these patients. The function of the single ventricle needs to be followed closely as well as the presence of leaking of the tricuspid valve. Some patients may have palpitations from rhythm disorders in the heart that may require medical therapy.

Medical advances to watch for: Treatments for rhythm disorders are improving. Other advances include improved techniques for cardiac transplantation and mechanical devices to help the ventricle pump more strongly.

PATENT DUCTUS ARTERIOSUS (PDA)

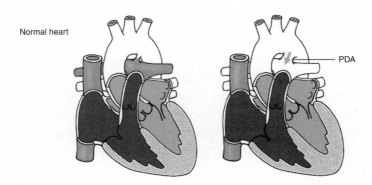

Normal heart

PDA

Name of defect: Patent ductus arteriosus (PDA)

Definition/anatomy: In utero, the ductus arteriosus is a large vessel that brings the fetus's blood to the lower body, bypassing the lungs, since the placental blood receives all the oxygen it needs from the mother. By the first week of life, the ductus arteriosus usually closes. If this vessel remains open, or patent, it is called a patent ductus arteriosus (PDA). When a large PDA is present, the left ventricle has to work harder to deal with the extra blood flow. A PDA is very common in premature babies.

Possible symptoms: Because blood flow to the aorta is returning to the left side of the heart, the left ventricle has to work harder than usual. Some infants may have symptoms of heart failure such as labored breathing, profuse sweating, and failure to grow.

Physical exam: Most infants and children with a PDA will have a prominent heart murmur.

Prognosis: Excellent. Coil closure in both the cardiac catheterization laboratory and surgery have excellent results. If the PDA is very large, surgical closure is the more likely option.

Treatment and surgical options: The PDA is closed either at surgery or in the cardiac catheterization laboratory. During surgery, the ductus is separated and tied off on each end. In the catheterization laboratory, a coil is placed in the ductus arteriosus that causes blood to thicken in that area and prevent further blood flow. Premature infants may be treated initially with a medicine called indomethacin, which, in some cases, causes the PDA to close without requiring an invasive procedure.

Surgical timing: Premature infants who have symptoms of heart failure should be treated initially with indomethacin. If this medical therapy isn't successful, they must be treated surgically. Older infants and children should be treated directly with either surgical intervention or catheter intervention.

Medications and medical care presurgery: These children need prophylactic antibiotics before dental surgery, since they're at risk for infection at the site of the ductus. In fact, most serious complications in childhood and infancy result from such infection. If an infant or child has significant heart failure, he or she may need medical therapy such as digoxin and furosemide immediately prior to a closure procedure.

Medications and medical care postsurgery: Medical care includes routine postoperative care in an ICU for one or two days. No specific medical therapy is necessary after surgery.

Possible restrictions: None.

Long-term concerns: The vast majority of patients require no long-term follow-up. Rarely, after surgical or transcatheter closure of a PDA, it can reopen a number of years later. In these cases, if the blood flow is significant across the ductus, reclosure may be indicated. Prophylactic antibiotics are recommended for six months after closure in the catheterization laboratory, but is no longer necessary after successful surgical closure.

Medical advances to watch for: Further advancements of transcatheter closure of large PDAs are in development.

STENOTIC PULMONARY VALVE

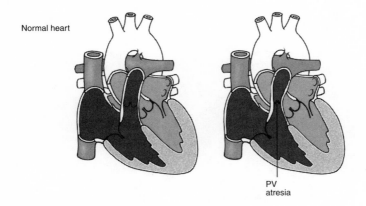

Normal heart

PV
atresia

Name of defect: Stenotic valves

Definition/anatomy: There are four valves in the heart: two on the right side—the tricuspid and pulmonic valves—and two on the left side—the mitral and aortic valves. These valves can be narrow at birth or become narrowed later in life.

Pulmonic valve stenosis: Narrowing of the pulmonic valve can range from mild to severe, in which the valve is completely closed (valve atresia). If the opening is very tiny, serious complications can re-

STENOTIC AORTIC VALVE

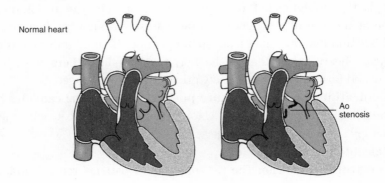

sult. In these cases, the valve should be opened urgently, most often by balloon dilatation.

Aortic valve stenosis: When the aortic valve is narrow, the left ventricle has to work harder to pump the blood to the rest of the body. Generally, the more narrow the valve, the harder the ventricle has to work and the more likely the infant or child will have symptoms such as low blood pressure and heart failure. Balloon dilatation and/or surgery may be required.

STENOTIC MITRAL VALVE

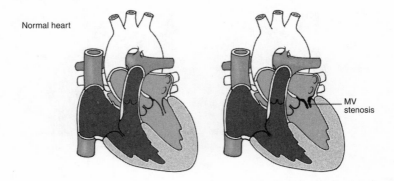

Mitral valve stenosis: Several different congenital malformations can lead to a narrowing of the mitral valve. If the narrowing is significant, heart failure can result. If the valve is completely closed at birth, it is called hypoplastic left heart syndrome (see page 44).

Tricuspid valve stenosis: If the tricuspid valve is very small, the right ventricle is also likely to be very small, and there may be no pulmonary valve opening. This type of congenital defect would require complex surgery for palliation (Fontan procedure).

STENOTIC TRICUSPID VALVE

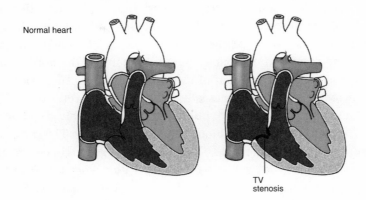

Normal heart

TV
stenosis

Possible symptoms: The symptoms vary depending on which valve is stenotic and how severe the narrowing is.

Pulmonic valve stenosis: If the valve is only mildly narrowed, the child may have no symptoms. However, if the valve is severely narrowed, the child may be cyanotic and have shortness of breath. Infants may require urgent intervention in the cardiac catheterization laboratory to relieve the obstruction. Pulmonic valve atresia is associated with complex congenital heart disease. These infants often have cyanosis within the first few days or weeks of life and require early surgery to connect the right ventricle to the pulmonary artery. A connection from the subclavian artery to the pulmonary artery (Blalock-Taussig shunt) is usually performed at the same time.

Aortic valve stenosis: Children with mild narrowing will have few or no symptoms. If the valve causes significant obstruction to blood flow, infants and children can have symptoms of congestive heart failure.

Mitral valve stenosis: If narrowing of the mitral valve is significant, infants and children can have symptoms of congestive heart failure. Older children will have shortness of breath with exertion.

Prognosis: Prognosis for valvular stenosis is generally very good. In most cases these valves can be opened in the cardiac catheterization laboratory. In some cases surgical correction is required.

Treatment and surgical options: Most forms of valvular stenosis can be opened with a dilating balloon in the catheterization laboratory. The possible side effect of this treatment is leaking from the valve, also called "valvular regurgitation," following the procedure. This leaking must be monitored, as it is possible that the valves will need to be replaced in the future if the leaking unduly strains the heart. Leaking of the aortic valve is more of a concern than leaking of the pulmonic valve, although both may require correction if the heart becomes very enlarged or has difficulty pumping in the increased amount of blood. Opening of the aortic valve does not last as long as treatment of the pulmonic valve. The procedure must be repeated a number of years later if the narrowing returns.

Sometimes surgery is the best option to fix the valve. Valves can be replaced with either mechanical or bioprosthetic (pig) valves. The valve size will depend on the size of the child. Generally the surgeon will choose the largest possible valve to delay the need for reoperation when the heart outgrows its replacement valve. For severe aortic stenosis, many centers advocate using the patient's own pulmonary valve (pulmonary autograft) in the aortic position, with a homograft (cadaverous) in the pulmonary position (Ross operation).

Surgical timing: The timing of surgery depends on the degree of stenosis of the valve and the amount of strain on the heart. Echocardiograms, electrocardiograms, and cardiac catheterizations can help the cardiologist decide if it is time to fix a valve.

Medications and medical care presurgery: If the narrowed valve has led to heart failure or swelling in the arms or belly, then medications such as furosemide, which is a diuretic, may be prescribed. In those cases, however, it is best to fix the valve itself. Prophylactic antibiotics therapy is needed before dental procedures to prevent endocarditis.

Medications and medical care postsurgery: If a valve is replaced with a mechanical prosthesis, then a blood-thinning medication called warfarin will be prescribed. Warfarin helps prevent clots from forming on the mechanical valve. It is very important to monitor the levels of warfarin in the blood because high levels may result in bleeding. Prophylactic antibiotics are needed before dental procedures.

Possible restrictions: If the valve is opened with a balloon in the catheterization lab, no specific restrictions apply. If, however, the valve is replaced and the patient is treated with warfarin, then he or she should avoid contact sports and heavy weight lifting.

Long-term concerns: If a child is treated with a mechanical valve, he or she will have to take warfarin for life. Warfarin may pose some risk to developing fetuses. Therefore, pregnant women will have to communicate closely with their cardiologists. Research is under way to find out what, if any, is the safest dose of warfarin for pregnant women. Some physicians prefer to replace warfarin with another medicine during pregnancy.

Aortic stenosis, which is treated in the cardiac catheterization laboratory, needs to be monitored carefully for either the degree of leaking after the catheterization or for recurrence of the narrowing.

Medical advances to watch for: Several new types of valves have been developed over recent years. There remains interest in the use of homograft valves, which don't require warfarin and could last up to fifteen years or more without needing replacement.

TETRALOGY OF FALLOT

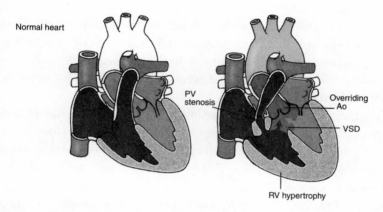

Normal heart

PV stenosis

Overriding Ao

VSD

RV hypertrophy

Name of defect: Tetralogy of Fallot

Definition/anatomy: Tetralogy of Fallot is a malformation of the heart that has four components:

1. Narrowing of the pulmonary valve
2. A large VSD
3. A dilated aorta that is connected to both the right and the left ventricles
4. Hypertrophy (thickening) of the right ventricle (This thickening results from the right ventricle having to work harder to pass blood across the narrowed pulmonary valve and into the lungs.)

Possible symptoms in infants: Infants with very severe narrowing of the pulmonary valve will have symptoms of cyanosis such as blue discoloration of the lips and nails, developing before one year of age. Occasionally infants between two and nine months of age will have sudden episodes of very rapid breathing. During these periods they may also have more intense blue discoloration of their fingers and lips. These "spells" occur most commonly in the morning after awakening and can be very serious. Placing the infant's knees up to his or her chest is helpful. The pediatric cardiologist should be notified during or immediately after such an event. Medical therapies used for this condition are oxygen and morphine, which help by increasing blood flow to the lungs.

If the pulmonary valve narrowing is less severe, the child will appear relatively normal. Rarely, an infant will show symptoms similar to those of a large VSD (difficulty feeding, excessive sweating, and failure to thrive).

Possible symptoms in children: Many children will naturally assume a squatting position after exercise as a way to increase pulmonary blood flow. Some may complain of shortness of breath or show blue discoloration of lips and fingers after exercise.

Prognosis: The prognosis for tetralogy of Fallot is very good. The surgical treatment has been well established. In some infants, the vessels in the lungs may be smaller than normal. In these cases the surgery is more complicated because graft material needs to be added to the arteries in the lungs to make the arteries larger.

Treatment and surgical options: The surgical treatment for tetralogy of Fallot involves two steps. A patch is used to close the hole between the left and the right ventricle, and the pulmonary valve narrowing is relieved. Over time, the right ventricle will become less thick and more normal in size.

Surgical timing: Surgery is now being performed safely on young infants. The timing often depends on how large the vessels are in the lungs. If these vessels are large enough to give the infant the oxygen he or she needs, then surgery can wait until the baby is larger and stronger. If the vessels are small, than a preliminary surgery called a Blalock-Taussig shunt may be done before full corrective surgery is performed later. This procedure involves redirecting some of the blood supplying the right or the left arm to one of the vessels in the lungs.

Medications and medical care presurgery: Generally, patients need no medicines before surgical repair of this defect.

Medications and medical care postsurgery: In rare cases, patients may need medical therapy for a few months after surgery. Occasionally heart rhythm disturbances occur that may require treatment.

Possible restrictions: After surgery for tetralogy of Fallot, children may not be able to exercise as vigorously as other children. Generally, they should avoid extreme forms of athletic activities.

Long-term concerns: When the narrowing of the pulmonary valve is relieved, there is often a considerable amount of leaking left in its place. Generally this leaking has few consequences. However, occasionally, over many years, the right ventricle may enlarge and the pulmonary valve may need to be replaced.

Some of these patients develop abnormal heart rhythms in the right ventricle. Generally these rhythms cause no ill effects, but the cardiologist will most likely have to follow up with routine tests such as electrocardiograms (EKGs) and Holter monitors.

Medical advances to watch for: Pulmonary valve replacements are being investigated in the cardiac catheterization laboratory. This procedure would avoid the necessity of a repeat operation in those patients who require a new pulmonary valve.

TOTAL ANOMALOUS PULMONARY VENOUS RETURN

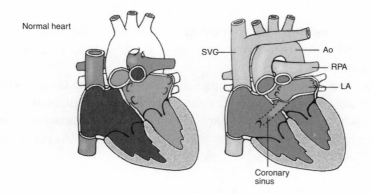

Name of defect: Total anomalous pulmonary venous return (TAPV)

Definition/anatomy: In a normal heart, the blood supply to the lungs returns to the left side of the heart via four distinct pulmonary veins that drain into the left atrium. In TAPV, the pulmonary veins drain abnormally to the right atrium through a common pulmonary vein. Blood is then supplied to the left side of the heart through a small hole (patent foramen ovale or atrial septal defect) in the wall that separates the left and the right atria.

Possible symptoms: Symptoms depend primarily on whether the anomalous pulmonary veins are obstructed.

If blood flow is severely obstructed, the infant will show symptoms shortly after birth or within the first few days of life. Symptoms include cyanosis (blue baby) and congestive heart failure (rapid breathing and failure to thrive). If less obstruction is present, the infant will show such symptoms after the first few months of life. If there is no obstruction to flow, symptoms will be mild or nonexistent. The child may later develop the same symptoms of a large atrial septal defect (see page 38).

Prognosis: Excellent after successful surgery.

Treatment and surgical options: The surgery for this defect involves reconnecting the pulmonary vein flow to the left atrium. Often tissue from around the heart (pericardial tissue) is used to make this connection.

Surgical timing: All patients with this defect should have corrective surgery as soon as possible after the diagnosis is made.

Medications and medical care presurgery: Sometimes an intravenous medication (Prostaglandin E1) is used to keep the connection between the aorta and the pulmonary artery (ductus arteriosus) open prior to surgery. Some infants with significant heart failure may need a breathing machine before surgery.

Medications and medical care postsurgery: Infants and children will need to stay in a specialized intensive care unit for several days after surgery.

Possible restrictions: No restrictions of physical activity are necessary after successful corrective surgery. Prophylactic antibiotics are needed before dental procedures.

Long-term concerns: Narrowing can develop either at the site where the pulmonary veins are sutured to the left atrium or within the veins themselves. Occasionally infants or children can develop abnormal heart rhythms originating from the upper chambers of the heart. All children will need careful follow-up with a pediatric cardiologist.

TRANSPOSITION OF THE GREAT VESSELS

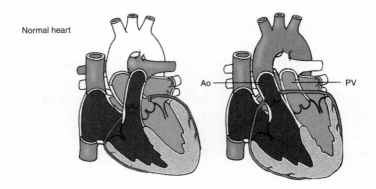

Normal heart

Ao   PV

Name of defect: Transposition of the great vessels (TGV)

Definition/anatomy: This malformation involves a reversal of the pulmonary artery and the aorta, resulting in abnormal blood flow. Blood normally flows from the right side of the heart to the lungs, to the left side of the heart, throughout the body, and back to the right side of the heart. In infants with TGV, blood flows from the right side of the heart to the body and back to the right side of the heart. Simultaneously, blood flows from the left side of the heart to the lungs and back to the left side of the heart. Prior to recent advances both in the cardiac catheterization laboratory and at surgery, the prognosis for this disease was grim. Currently, however, the outlook for properly managed infants and children is excellent.

Possible symptoms: Infants born with transposition of the great vessels are cyanotic ("blue baby"). The amount of cyanosis depends on whether there are associated lesions that cause mixing of blood from the right and the left circulation, usually through the two atria. However, virtually all newborns with this diagnosis need immediate treatment.

Prognosis: The prognosis for this disease is now excellent, given the rapid advances in surgical treatment.

Treatment and surgical options: The surgery of choice in these patients is the arterial switch procedure placing the aorta in its correct position attached to the left ventricle and placing the pulmonary artery in its correct position attached to the right ventricle. During this procedure, the coronary arteries that provide blood to the heart muscle are switched from the pulmonary artery to the aorta.

Surgical timing: The arterial switch procedure is almost always done right after birth.

Medications and medical care presurgery: Directly after birth, some infants require a procedure in the catheterization laboratory that involves taking a balloon and opening a hole in the wall between the two atria. This allows oxygen to perfuse the body and brain until full corrective surgery can be done.

Medications and medical care postsurgery: After surgery, patients require care in a specialized intensive care unit. A typical hospital stay after surgery is seven to ten days.

Possible restrictions: No restrictions apply after successful corrective repair.

Long-term concerns: Because the coronary arteries are "reimplanted" into the aorta from the pulmonary artery, it is possible that they may be injured. It is still unknown if these patients will have a higher risk of coronary artery disease later in life. Studies are under way to investigate this possibility, but only a few patients followed through adolescence have been found to have serious coronary abnormalities.

Medical advances to watch for: New ways to assess the coronary arteries that don't require cardiac catheterization are rapidly developing. These techniques include magnetic resonance imaging (MRI) and ultrafast CT scanning.

VENTRICULAR SEPTAL DEFECT (VSD)

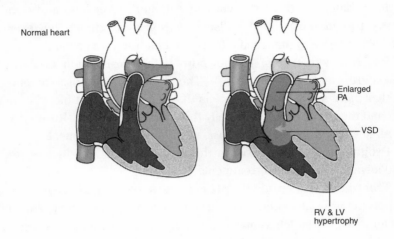

Normal heart

Enlarged PA

VSD

RV & LV hypertrophy

Name of defect: Ventricular septal defect (VSD)

Definition/anatomy: A VSD is a hole or opening between the right and the left ventricles. It may be very small, in which case surgery isn't necessary. The majority of these VSDs become smaller or even close on their own. If the VSD is large, the left side of heart will have to pump harder because it is supplying the blood to the entire body and at the same time back into the lungs via the right ventricle. This extra workload may lead to heart failure. In addition, the extra blood flow to the lungs can lead to lung disease. Therefore, all large VSDs should be closed surgically. The best treatment for a medium-sized VSD is less clear. In general these cases can be followed medically because they may become smaller or occasionally close.

Possible symptoms: Infants show symptoms of heart failure (difficulty feeding, excessive sweating, failure to grow). Older children experience shortness of breath with exertion.

Prognosis: Excellent. This defect is very amenable to surgical correction.

Treatment and surgical options: A patch is sewn over the opening between the left and the right ventricles.

Surgical timing: The timing depends on the size of the hole. Large VSDs should be closed within the first eighteen months of life.

Medications and medical care presurgery: In infancy, the presurgical care will depend on whether the baby has heart failure, in which case digitalis and furosemide are used.

Medications and medical care postsurgery: Once the VSD is closed and the heart has recovered, long-term medications are not necessary. Prophylactic antibiotics to prevent endocarditis are needed for only the first six months after surgery. Once the patch has healed and no residual shunt is present, no antibiotic pretreatment for dental work is necessary.

Possible restrictions: If the defect is small or has been surgically closed, the child has no restrictions on physical activity.

Long-term concerns: VSDs that aren't fully closed require prophylactic antibiotics before dental procedures. Long-term complications are extremely rare.

Medical advances to watch for: Closure of VSDs by catheterization may become available for certain cases.

CHAPTER 3

COPING

Dennis Sklenar, C.S.W.   Jonathan Slater, M.D.

Y OUR child's been diagnosed. You've started learning about CHD. Now, how do you cope while you wait for something to be done about it?

Some children will go right from delivery to the neonatal intensive care unit. That must be especially hard, because you don't have time alone—at home—with your newborn. The hospital becomes your home, and your difficult times are often spent in the midst of a lot of strangers.

Not all cases will require surgery, and not all cases will require surgery right away. Many families are given the tough task of going about normal life with an unrepaired CHD looming, waiting to see if it will go away or if medicine will solve the problem, or waiting for the right time to schedule surgery.

Besides watching for signs of heart problems, we were learning to care for our first baby. Was he eating enough? Why did nursing hurt so much? Why did he throw up all that milk—again? We were on the phone to our cardiologist and our pediatrician all the time. We even had our cardiologist's home number.

Ours was not a "pass-around" baby, and visits to the cardiologist were not easy. We would literally spend hours there, trying to keep Max calm so the doctor could get good EKG readings and echos. I nursed Max before and during many tests and procedures to keep him calm.

When Max was born, the doctor thought he'd need heart surgery at about three or four months of age. Or maybe later. Then, with each checkup, they'd put the pulse oximeter on his finger or toe, and the number would be lower (and scarier). Or they'd do an echo, and the pulmonary artery would be narrower. With each checkup, things got more serious, and it looked like our trip to the hospital would be sooner than expected. This was no easy task, living day to day, waiting for the word on when we would have to go. And the fact that we lived in Roanoke, Virginia, and would have to go out of town for surgery—a four-hour drive away—made it more difficult. Finally, we were told to go. Definitive action. However horrifying the thought of surgery was, it was a relief to be getting it over with. Then, more ambivalence. We were told there was the chance they'd examine him at the hospital and decide to put off the surgery. They didn't put off the surgery. All thoughts that we would wake up from our nightmare vanished the day we were admitted. This was for real. Max was three and a half weeks old.

Gerri

Sharing the News

How do I tell people about my baby's defect? I want them to see my baby as a person, not a "condition."

Dr. Slater: I would be selective about whom you tell concerning your baby's condition. Close friends and family can be told as you feel comfortable, but decide for yourself how much questioning and "checking up on" you welcome. Some people prefer the close support and involvement of others, and some find it intrusive. Whatever your level of comfort, communicate this to the people you tell, and who ask about your child. If you do tell others about it, I would do so matter-of-factly, emphasizing that this is something that will be treated, and not dwelling on it too much. This way you'll give the implicit message that your baby isn't defined by the condition.

TELLING FRIENDS AND FAMILY

"We told the news mostly through a communication chain. We really didn't want to talk about it over and over."

—*Lisa Kay Hartmann, mom to Jenna*
(*tetralogy of Fallot with pulmonary atresia*)

"Telling people was initially very difficult—I would break down in tears. After a while, I stuck to the medical facts and tried to keep my emotions out of it."

—*Jean Buerle Farley, nurse, and mom to Colleen*
(*critical pulmonary stenosis*)

"Zachary was diagnosed with his heart defects while I was still in the hospital with him. The whole thing is very overwhelming. People don't want to call because they don't know what to say. Family keeps asking questions that you can't answer. People stopped sending flowers and cards. After a while I didn't even want to pick up the phone so I had my friend answer it for me. It was so hard repeating things that I was barely comprehending."

—*Carole Stoll, mom to Zachary*
(VSD, subaortic stenosis, interrupted aortic arch)

"We told everyone about Alex's condition. Knowing that there were people in several states praying for us as Alex underwent his surgeries and recovered from them was a comfort and relieved us from shouldering the entire emotional burden."

—*Sara Daniel, mom to Alex (tricuspid atresia, ASD, VSD)*

"We have had so many people dismiss it (which is annoying) or go to the other extreme (oh, poor, poor girl—what a miracle baby, etc.), which is just as annoying if not more so."

—*Diane and Trent Barilko, parents of Alexandra (double outlet right*
ventricle, pulmonary atresia with a VSD, discontinuous LPA, major
aorto/pulmonary collateral arterials, pulmonary branch stenosis)

"People ask a lot of questions and sometimes say the wrong things. . . . Try to remember that you probably didn't know much about CHD before your child had it."

—*Roberta Love, mom to Allison (ventricular inversion,*
double outlet left ventricle, rudimentary right ventricle,
transposition of the great arteries, VSD)

How do I tell my older children? What's the best way to do it without scaring them too much?

Dr. Slater: This depends on the age of the older children. School-age (six to twelve years) children can look at pictures from books or pamphlets. As calmly as you can, tell them that their sister or brother was born with a problem in the heart (you may need to explain what the heart is first!) that makes the blood not flow properly. You can explain in simple terms what the doctors have planned and show it in a diagram. You'll find books on the body for children of all ages in your local library or bookstore. I would emphasize that this is *not* a problem they were born with, can develop, or "catch." Assure them that their sibling is receiving the best care, that he or she is healthy in every other respect (assuming this is true), and should be fine.

EXPLAINING CHD TO SIBLINGS

"We bought our older boys (six and four) an anatomy book and we showed them where the problem was and how it was fixed. We drew many pictures."

—Jane Beard, mom to Evan
(coarctation of the aorta, valve defect, missing coronary artery)

"We told our other daughter that her sister's heart was 'broken' and a doctor was going to fix it. She thought the baby's incision was like a zipper to open her chest and fix her heart."

—Susan Wirth, nurse and mom to Julie (interrupted aortic arch, VSD, ASD)

"We have always told both of our children that our second child had a 'special' heart that worked differently from the rest of ours. Before his second and third surgeries, we told them both that the doctors were going to make his heart work better so he wouldn't get tired so quickly."

—Joanne Baldauf, mom to Kenny (double inlet left ventricle with
outflow chamber and transposition of the great vessels)

"Our older son seems to have a lot of insight into complex issues, so we have always been very straightforward and honest in explaining Andrew's defect with him. He understands that Andrew was born with his heart not working properly and that the doctors had to open him up to fix his heart, hence the scar. He's drawn simple pictures of the heart and pretends to 'lecture' about it."

—Alisa Spaulding, mom to Andrew (pulmonary atresia)

"I didn't think that it was affecting my three-year-old son. I should have paid more attention to him. I didn't realize that the situation was bothering him. We should have sat down and explained it all to him. He was very sad and didn't understand what was happening to his little brother."

—Mary Lisa Detterline, mom to Matthew (transposition, ASD, VSD)

"Before one of Zachary's surgeries, Melissa asked us if he was going to die. We reassured her that he wasn't, but I know she heard the uncertainty in my words. You don't realize how much the older children pick up from hearing you talk on the phone and from knowing you well enough to tell that you are nervous."

—Carole Stoll, mom to Zachary
(VSD, subaortic stenosis, interrupted aortic arch)

We have a party planned to celebrate my baby's birth and I feel funny celebrating. Is it okay to celebrate, even though he has a heart defect?

Dr. Slater: Of course it's okay! You're celebrating the birth of your child, and you deserve this. Your new baby is a person whom you loved from the moment you felt him inside you, and will grow to cherish from the moment of birth. Celebrate the life you created!

Is there anything I can tell people when they ask me how they can help me?

Dr. Slater: This depends on whether you think the particular person *can* help you. If not, you may appreciate the offer and say so, but assure them that you're doing okay. Otherwise, be specific. If there are ways they can help (anything from driving to baby-sitting to shopping), and you think the person's offer is genuine, go ahead and ask.

HOW OTHERS CAN HELP

"We found family and friends to be the best support. They took care of everything for us (during Kevin's surgery) so we could just concentrate on our child. We had both sets of grandparents come—each for a two-week period—to care for our other kids; that was a huge relief. Friends took turns making dinner for us, which also was great. We only talked to one person at our house and they relayed the information to other friends and relatives."

—Anne Linne, mom to Kevin (transposition of the great vessels)

"Our closest friends are involved like the family, but other friends do hesitate to call or come over in fear of the unknown. They don't know what to expect and are also afraid to ask."

—Dawn Howie, mom to Travis (HLHS)

"I would advise you to talk to a close friend or family member. Talking always helps me. Also, don't be afraid to cry."

—Shelly Corush, mom to Seth (coarctation of the aortic artery, enlarged pulmonary artery, several ASDs and VSDs, heart block with a pacemaker—as a result of the ASD and VSD repair surgery)

"Time, helping with the siblings, cooking, laundry, especially when the child is hospitalized, taking turns at the hospital to give parents a break. Blood donations, a shoulder to cry on—a sounding board. Many cards and letters and drawings from the kids' friends for the child in the hospital."

—Joanne Baldauf, mom to Kenny (double inlet left ventricle with outflow chamber and transposition of the great vessels)

"The best support from others is listen, listen, listen."

—Sylvia Paul, mom to Alyssa (tricuspid atresia)

"During surgery: Take up the 'watch' while the parents go to the hospital cafeteria for a meal. Hold their hand. Physical contact is important. Day-to-day: Let the parents know that you understand they are concerned for their child, and don't belittle their concerns about their child's health."

—Sue Dove, mom to Scott (single ventricle)

"I think one of the best things they can do is listen and try not to trivialize things. They need to understand that what seems to be a minor illness in other children can cause major problems for a heart child and that just because a heart child may look like there's nothing wrong doesn't mean that nothing can ever go wrong again."

—Lou Anne Wright, mom to Nicole (transposition of the great arteries)

"Instead of downplaying or even outright ignoring our worries and fears, family and friends can offer an understanding ear to our concerns. At the very least they can refrain from making comments such as 'Why do you still have concerns about Andrew's heart if he's fixed now?' "

—Alisa Spaulding, mom to Andrew (pulmonary atresia)

"An offer like 'You take care of the sick child and we will take care of the others when you need us to. . . . Don't worry, we will help' is wonderful because surgery/hospitalization requires complete devotion to the sick child."

—Karen Dahlman, mom to Rebecca (ASD)

I want to tell people about my baby's heart problem, but I feel terribly embarrassed. What's the best way to approach this?

Dr. Slater: Ask yourself what you are embarrassed about. It isn't your fault, and it's nothing to be ashamed about. Generally people react with sensitivity and tact, given the feelings naturally evoked in people when they hear that a baby has a problem. No one will judge you.

What's the best approach to tell others in my workplace about my daughter's heart condition?

Dr. Slater: Most parents worry that they will be closely scrutinized and that others will fear that they will not be able to complete their responsibilities. In fact, people in the workplace are generally understanding, and a parent has a right to take a medical leave from work. It's better to be honest with employers, since a sick child understandably can affect job attendance and performance, and it's best for them to know what is going on. This will also allow them to lend a helping hand, or make temporary arrangements to give you assistance at work.

How do I tell my boss that I will need to take time off from work? How much notice will I be able to give him?

Mr. Sklenar: Dr. Slater's comment about telling other people about your baby's defect holds true about informing your boss. However, it's important to give your boss all of the facts, and to be up front regarding what you feel you will need. Sometimes a letter from the physician is helpful giving many of the details, and makes your request for time off more legitimate to the boss. Most employers are understanding and sensitive to these issues, and may allow you to use vacation and sick days. How much notice you will have to give depends upon your baby's medical condition and the employer. The Family Leave Act enables you to take unpaid leave to care for a sick family member without jeopardizing your position. Check with your employer about the details, as paperwork will need to be filed.

A GRANDPARENT'S PERSPECTIVE
By Joel Freid, Ph.D., clinical psychologist

At a family gathering in November 1994, our daughter and son-in-law took my wife and me aside to give us the most exciting news we could ever wish for. Gerri, our daughter, was pregnant—her first child, our first grandchild. I recall some of the same feelings of joy, pride, and excitement I had felt some thirty-odd years before when I came home to the news that Ellie, my wife, was pregnant with Gerri—our first child.

Gerri immediately began reading everything she could find about pregnancy, childbirth, and child rearing. She was a careful, healthy eater, never smoked, and never drank alcohol during her pregnancy. She was preparing to give birth to the "perfect child." Intellectually, we all knew that there always could be some problem, but for me that no-tion was easily dismissed. After all, Ellie and I were blessed with three healthy, perfect children. When Max was born with a congenital heart defect that would require nearly immediate surgery, it was, to say the least, a shock.

I was in Florida and my wife was in Virginia with our children when Max was born. Ellie called with the good news. I was elated, excited, and very proud—a grandson! I called some other relatives with the good news and went out and bought an IT'S A BOY streamer to hang in my office. The next day, while I was on my way over to hang a streamer in my wife's office, she called to tell me that the doctor had heard a heart murmur in Max and that he might have a heart defect. At that point he hadn't been examined by a cardiologist, so she couldn't share a lot of information with me. I remember that my own heart dropped then, and all my joy and excitement turned to fear and confusion. I also recall that this period of waiting and not knowing exactly what the problem was was one of the most difficult times I have ever endured.

Another memory stands out from that day. Bringing the streamer into my wife's office, by chance I ran into a close friend of ours. She asked if the baby had been born yet, and with the best smile and happy tone I could muster I proclaimed, "Oh, yes, it's a boy, Max, and he's beautiful and everybody's doing fine." Knowing my friend, I was sure that she could sense the incongruence between the words coming out of my mouth and the expression on my face. However, I was in no mood—nor was I well-enough informed—to discuss it further. Angry that I could not report the birth of that long-awaited perfect child, I left the office crying.

Feeling helpless and afraid, I decided to call a pediatrician friend of mine and share with him the little bit of information I did have about Max. He took time and gently talked with me about congenital heart defects—a conversation that was immeasurably important at that time, not only for the information, but also for the reassurance and support. Although I still had many questions and much anxiety, I felt a sense of comfort and hope.

The day after Max was born, Ellie returned to the hospital and found Gerri's room empty. Ellie was very scared. It turned out Max had just been examined by the pediatric cardiologist. Our children were obviously upset. Max was diagnosed with tetralogy of Fallot. Shaken and in disbelief, my wife still wanted to be strong for the children. But she hardly knew what the next step should be. She still remembers the frightened look on our children's faces and not being sure how to comfort them. How hard it must have been to call me with the news, hear the unhappiness in my voice! How helpless I felt being so far away. For me at that point there were many tears, much anxiety, and a terrible feeling of being out of control of my life.

At that point, the doctors didn't think that Max's condition was too serious. Gerri and Jeff left the hospital with Max and some cautionary notes about how long he should be allowed to cry, and keeping an eye on his color. Once home, however, they weren't sure what was normal and what was not.

A week later I flew to Virginia. When I arrived, the children were at the doctor's office with Max. I recall my wife and I were sitting on the front porch hours later when they returned. We watched them pull up and park across the street. We watched as our daughter got out of the car holding Max in his carrier and broke down and cried. We learned that Max would need surgery within weeks. Now we were torn between fears of Max's condition and fears of the surgery required to hopefully make it better.

At the ripe old age of three and a half weeks, Max had open-heart surgery. We cheer this amazingly strong little boy and his brave parents, who insisted they could manage on their own, and that they did. We spoke to them frequently by telephone and got regular progress reports, but there was always that fear of the unknown, feelings of helplessness from a distance—we wanted to do something, but frankly we didn't know what to do except pray.

As a clinical psychologist, I have counseled numerous families of children born with serious health problems—developmental disabilities, congenital defects, chronic life-threatening illnesses, and others. It is well documented that the emotional impact on parents who have a child born with a defect or a disability can be overwhelming—even devastating at times. Parents report being in shock, a state of disbelief, as in "this can't be happening to us." Spousal conflict, guilt, self-blame, and self-pity complicate these matters of life and death. The research suggests that in some cases, mothers of children born with congenital defects may be afraid to get too close to their child for fear that the child will die. With the best of intentions, they draw back at a time when attachment is vital. Other parents become overprotective. Parents report a myriad of emotions, including fear, anger, worry, guilt, shame—and overwhelming sadness. This is a time for crying, for mourning the lost dream of having a healthy child. Many authors have stressed the importance of this mourning period, which eventually, thankfully, gives way to acceptance and adaptation. Not only the mother and father, but also the siblings, grandparents, aunts, and uncles mourn in their own ways.

The failure to provide families with the information, support, and counseling they need to understand their child's condition may cause more pain, anxiety, and confusion than the condition itself. As human beings we are all inherently strong, but also very vulnerable when an unexpected event such as the birth of an unhealthy child occurs. Prompt, straightforward, complete, and accurate medical information is crucial, as are counseling, reassurance, and realistic hope. Often parents need to talk—especially with other people in similar circumstances. Support groups and now communication via the Internet make it easier.

Max's surgery was a success. Despite his problems at birth, he is indeed our perfect grandchild. As I come to the end of this story, my eyes are swimming with tears, not of sorrow but of thanks for Max's life and the joy he brings to ours. When I hold him, see his smile, or just hear him say the word "grandpa," he fills my heart with strength. When I see Max I never think of him as being unhealthy or anything less than normal—he's Max, he's extraordinary, the smartest one in his class, the best soccer player on his team. He can name every team in the NFL, throw a ball straight as an arrow, and be the most loving little child—just ask him—or better yet, just ask his grandparents.

Discussing CHD with Your Child

My five-year-old was just diagnosed with CHD. Do I tell him? If so, how? How do I tell a toddler? What about a preteen?

Dr. Slater: I would get some picture books appropriate to a five-year-old, or stuffed animals with organs (special companies make these, and Child Life departments often have them), and explain quite simply what the problem is, stressing how it will be fixed. A toddler can understand that he is sick and the doctors are making him better if you use appropriate terms such as "boo-boo inside," pointing to the chest. A preteen can follow more complicated diagrams and direct (but still optimistic) explanations. Preteens also can question doctors themselves.

"When I talk to Scott, I tell him that God must have made him like this for a reason. No two people are alike, some are short, some are tall, some have perfect hearts, some don't, some are blind, some can't hear, but God loves us all and wants us all to be the best person we can."

—*Sue Dove, mom to Scott (single ventricle)*

My child is old enough to understand everything. How do I prepare him for the hospital without scaring him? How soon before his surgery should I tell him that he will be having surgery?

Dr. Slater: You can prepare him by having him visit and tour the hospital, and by doing some "medical play" in which you simulate various aspects of the surgery. When you tell the child depends on the age, but generally several weeks are needed to prepare most children adequately. Not telling them until the last minute will make them more anxious, not less, especially about something unexpected happening in the future. Child Life specialists, psychologists, and psychiatrists with experience in this area can do this type of preparation in several visits. Tell your child you will be with him in the hospital, and that there will be medicine for the hurt. Don't mislead the child or misrepresent what will happen.

"Prepare your child for the hospital stay. Be as honest as possible with him or her. Don't minimize the event, but don't dwell on it either. More like 'You have to be fixed so we are going to get that taken care of so that you can be better.'"

—Sue Dove, mom to Scott (single ventricle)

My child had a surgical repair as an infant and currently has no restrictions. When is the right time to explain her defect to her, and what is the best way to do that?

Dr. Slater: As part of growing up, it's important to explain the past. As soon as a child is old enough to notice he or she has a scar, you can explain what happened, using appropriate books, drawings, and other props.

Finding Support

There must be other people going through this. How can I find them?

Dr. Slater: Internet support groups, organizations such as the American Heart Association, and departments of pediatric cardiology are all good resources. You can also ask your doctor for names of other families you could contact. (See the Resources section of this book for more information on support groups.)

"Try to get as much information in advance [of the surgery] as possible. Visit the ICU, look at pictures of kids after their surgery, search for information about your child's CHD. But most of all, meet with parents and kids who have undergone similar surgeries. Kids are so resilient that in just a few short weeks after surgery most are as active as ever. Just seeing that they look 'normal' and have survived such trauma can give parents (and their children) new hope. In addition, knowledge alleviates some fear."

—*Randy Sittner, dad to Isaiah*
(hypoplastic right ventricle, pulmonary atresia, and tricuspid atresia)

"Do research, become informed so you can make informed judgments because you are going to be called on to do that."

—*Pat Posada Klapper, mom to Alexandra (VSD)*

I looked on the Internet for information on my baby's heart defect. Some of the stories seemed very depressing and many had negative outcomes, but my doctor tells me my child will be fine. Who do I believe?

Dr. Slater: You can't necessarily extrapolate from something you read about to your own child: every situation is different. You should trust your own doctor, and discuss with him or her what you read about and what your concerns are. It is also quite acceptable to obtain a second opinion to help you feel confident you are doing the best for your child.

SPOTLIGHT ON ...
Sheri Berger
Congenital Heart Disease Resource Page

When Sheri Berger called her friend Mary in June 1995 to congratulate her on the birth of her daughter, Sheri was surprised to hear that all was not well. Five-day-old Amanda had been diagnosed with tetralogy of Fallot, and poor Mary was absolutely overwhelmed by all of the doctors and the information they were bombarding her with. So Mary took a step back and asked a few of her friends to do some research for her. She asked Sheri, then one of the few people she knew with easy Internet access, to see what she could find through this emerging medium.

Sheri first explored the database Lexis-Nexis, but everything she found was too technical, and much of it was very depressing. Then she started posting to some news groups. Pretty soon people started writing back, telling her about Web sites, a CHD newsletter called *Chaser*, the book *The Heart of a Child*, and many other resources. Sheri sorted through this information. About a month after Mary had asked her to help, Sheri was able to present her with a wealth of information that she could use to educate herself about Amanda's problem.

This left Sheri with an abundance of information about congenital heart disease. She wasn't quite sure what to do with it all, but then it struck her—she had been considering doing a personal home page— wouldn't this make a great one! She put up the first page, "The Heart Page," in the summer of 1995. Pretty soon she was getting five to ten responses a week. These responses ranged from medical questions (which she answers politely with a letter stating that she is not a doctor and cannot give medical advice), to information on other resources, books, hospitals, and Web sites (which are added as she updates the page), to thank yous from people all over the world who have been helped by the page (which is what keeps her going, even when her busy schedule barely permits her to update the page). What started as one long information page has evolved into "The Congenital Heart Disease Resource Page," (www.bamdad.com/sheri/) one of the finest resources for people with CHD, with more than sixteen different subcategories.

And Sheri's work has been recognized by others on the Internet. "The Congenital Heat Disease Resource Page" has been awarded many awards, including the ABC's of Parenting 5 Star Site Award and Healthy Way™ Best of the Web.

Sheri grew up in Los Angeles, where she now lives with her husband. She teaches math at Cal State Northridge and Los Angeles Valley College. She is still very close to Mary and to Amanda, who is six years old and doing fine. Little did they realize back in 1995 that Mary's call for help would be answered with one of the key resources for CHD.

SHERI BERGER'S TIPS ON USING THE INTERNET

1. Remember that the Internet is best used to find general information, not to make home diagnoses.
2. Read all disclaimers on medical sites.
3. Be wary of sites readily giving out medical advice. It is impossible for someone (even a qualified physician) to give a prognosis or recommend treatment without performing an examination.
4. Buyer beware! Information distributed on the Web may not be medically accurate.

5. When you find medical information on the Web, discuss it with your doctor.

6. Don't become overwhelmed. You'll likely turn up more information and personal stories than you can digest in a sitting. Take a break and discuss your concerns with people around you.

SUPPORT GROUPS AND THE INTERNET

"I have participated in two support groups. One of them is the PDHeart list on the Internet. The other is a group at our local children's hospital called "Heart to Heart." It is for parents of children with CHD. These groups are both very helpful to me. When I have questions I can come right to people who have been through my same situation. I love being part of our hospital's group because it keeps me familiar with being in the hospital, a place that can be kind of scary. The more you're there, the more comfortable you feel."
—*Deanna Smith, mom to Nicholas* (*HLHS*)

"Get into a support group at the onset and then, as you learn more and as the child gets older, you may no longer need it, but your child may benefit."
—*Sharon Popp, mom to Ben*
(*pulmonary atresia with VSD, transposition of the aorta*)

"I found the PDHeart listserve while doing research for this book and many members contributed to these pages. What I found remarkable about the group was the extent of the support and friendship that can develop over the Internet. Many among the group also arranged in-person get-togethers and exchanged holiday cards through the mail."
—*Gerri Kramer, mom to Max* (*tetralogy of Fallot*)

"I belong to PDHeart, which has been very helpful because support, information, and encouragement are at my fingertips."
—*Susie DeLoach, mom to Joey* (*HLHS*)

"We went on the Internet and found a lot of stuff we didn't want to read. We then got very concerned about Down syndrome, which is often associated with AV canal (Hannah does not have this) and worried a lot because I found so much information that didn't pertain to us."
—*Alex Rogers, dad to Hannah* (*AV canal*)

"I had a patient who was diagnosed with a heart defect. It was serious, but we were confident it could be repaired. However, the father went home that night and looked on the Internet and came back to me the next day furious— 'How could you give us hope when there is none?' He had gotten information on the Internet that wasn't accurate, but he thought we had given him the misinformation."

—Dr. Barbara Strassberg, pediatrician, Riverdale, New York

Living with CHD

What are some of the more common fears that parents confront after finding out their child has CHD? What questions should we be asking to ease our fears?

Dr. Slater: The most common fears involve whether the problem can be corrected, what the worst-case scenarios are, and how the baby's physical and intellectual growth will be affected. As well, there are often concerns about how to care for the baby outside the hospital (e.g., if nursing will be needed and/or possible), whether mothers will be able to work, and what the financial strains will be. Questions about the effects on siblings and marriages often arise. Parents should ask questions about all these things and take advantage of the multidisciplinary team that usually works with many pediatric cardiology departments. Write down your questions prior to visits and don't be too shy to ask every one of them.

Are there things we can do to make it easier to live with all of the risks associated with CHD?

Dr. Slater: Try to live as "normal" a life as possible. Parents still need time to themselves, both individually and together. Siblings still need attention and quality time with their parents. The family needs to have its fun and vacations. If you travel, discuss with your doctor beforehand what to do if a problem arises: where to go, whom to call, how to reach them. If monitoring equipment is needed, take it with you. Take advantage of vacation spots that cater to children, especially challenged children, if necessary (I have even written letters to Disney World in the past, so my patients wouldn't have to wait in lines). Pay attention to your own stress level as a parent, and that of your spouse and other children, and get counseling if you see signs or symptoms of excessive anxiety, depression, or stress.

COPING WITH CHD

"We don't talk about her defect much. Not because we're trying to hide it; we want it to be a natural part of her history, so we don't want to make too much of a big deal out of it. The only time we really think about it is when she needs to go to the dentist and take antibiotics."

—*Pat Posada Klapper, mom to Alexandra (VSD)*

"Even though he is corrected and seems fine, every day I think 'When is the other shoe going to drop? Will I lose my son?' I also experienced breathing problems and panic attacks within the year after his surgery. I am a big worrier, and everything snowballed. I finally got all of that under control with the help of a therapist."

—*Anne Linne, mom to Kevin (transposition of the great vessels)*

"I would have visions of being at his funeral. I felt like I was crazy, but I couldn't help it."

—*Carole Stoll, mom to Zachary*
(VSD, subaortic stenosis, interrupted aortic arch)

"God has a reason for giving you this special child to care for. Focus on the positive and look around you for the good things that will happen as a result of your experience. Don't let anger and bitterness toward God destroy you."

—*Sheryl Lamb, mom to Heather (double outlet right ventricle,*
hypoplastic right upper chamber, transposition,
subvalvular pulmonary stenosis, bilateral superior vena cava with
interrupted inferior vena cava, common ventricle)

"Hold on and have hope. There is a light at the end of the tunnel you feel like you're in. There is something very special in being able to raise a child who is a true miracle."

—*Susie DeLoach, mom to Joey (HLHS)*

How can I treat my child with the special care he needs without spoiling him?

Dr. Slater: You can separate the special requirements and limitations of a child with a medical condition from the expectations and roles a child is still able to fulfill. Don't let guilt over your child's condition and treatment prevent you from setting limits. Teach responsibility and respect for others, and the same values that you possess. Chores and responsibilities can be modified to let your child participate in ways he or she is able to manage.

"Because my son was cyanotic for some time and had so many procedures since birth, we had to limit his crying. We didn't want him *overly* excited. This produced a sometimes very whiny child. You have to balance a fine line between not wanting a bratty child and realizing that for good reason you have to keep him calm. Then, as soon as we got the okay from the cardiologist, it was time to let him cry and carry on more to sort of retrain him. It can be done, but it requires a lot of stamina!"

—Sharon Popp, mom to Ben
(pulmonary atresia with VSD, transposition of the aorta)

How do I avoid conflicts among my family when one child needs special care?

Dr. Slater: You can't. The situation is stressful for all involved, and conflicts are part of life both with and without a child with a medical condition; having a child with a medical condition presents a unique stress on a family, and conflicts are inevitable. Families with open lines of communication tend to adapt better, and professional help is often worthwhile.

CHD AND THE FAMILY

"I wish I had been better prepared for the stress that this caused on the rest of my family. When you have other children at home, it's very difficult to juggle everything. I'm not sure how I could have prepared for this, but I wasn't ready for it at all."

—Deanna Smith, mom to Nicholas (HLHS)

"Involving siblings in home treatment helps them feel important and included."
—Laurie Beard, mom to Trevor (tetralogy of Fallot, Down syndrome)

"I figure that this kind of thing is going to make or break relationships. Either you are in it together or not. I find that my already strong marriage has been strengthened by our united front in securing the best care possible for our son. Having said that, my husband and I feel differently at different times and we have had to learn how to accept the other person's emotional needs (or lack thereof) at times."

—Laurie Strongin, mom to Henry (tetralogy of Fallot)

"There has been stress placed on our marriage. Rick and I discovered, after talking with a marriage counselor, that we have some hidden anger about Joey's heart problem. We learned that it's deep down inside and kind of comes out 'sideways' at each other—that's part of the reason we were bickering about little things. We're learning to admit we have that anger and find other ways to channel it. We've learned it's okay to be mad at the defect, mad at God for giving it to him, and mad about what it does to us. She taught us that being mad at the defect has nothing to do with the way we feel about Joey, and we should teach him when he's older it's okay, even healthy, to express anger about it himself."

—Susie DeLoach, mom to Joey (HLHS)

"My older daughter, Melissa, looks at the time we spend with Zachary going to doctors, having tests, etc., as time we're spending with him and not her."

—Carole Stoll, mom to Zachary
(VSD, subaortic stenosis, interrupted aortic arch)

"We always made our son, Bobby, feel important, especially when Kelly was having surgery. We told him he was going to be an important part of our family 'supporting each other' through all of this."

—Maureen Goense, mom to Kelly (ASD)

"When our son was in the hospital, we kind of alternated going through bad times. I think we knew we both couldn't freak out. It was, however, very difficult for our other two children. They did not understand why we had to keep going to the hospital and why they couldn't hold the baby when he came home. Our older son, to this day, has very jealous feelings toward his brother. He has never understood the special treatment."

—Anne Linne, mom to Kevin (transposition of the great vessels)

"It was definitely stressful on our marriage before Josh's surgery, but we knew we could get through it. It made us stronger and even a little tougher."

—Rachael Beron, mom to Josh (tetralogy of Fallot)

My child is bright and inquisitive but very small for her age. Should I hold her back a grade in school so that she can be closer in size to her peers?

Dr. Slater: No. The decision to hold back a child should be based on developmental level, and social as well as cognitive capacity should be considered.

I need to go back to work in a few weeks. Is it okay to leave my baby with someone else?

Mr. Sklenar: This depends upon your baby's needs, and should be discussed in more detail with your physician. However, your baby's medical condition should not interfere with returning to work. Choose a mature, responsible, and trustworthy caretaker as you would in any case. Discuss medication schedules with your physician to see if you can take care of it early in the morning before you leave the house, or in the evening after you return. Inform your childcare provider completely about your baby's medical condition, and leave a list of any medications the baby is taking, instructions for how to reach you, and how to reach your physician's office. This person should also be advised on what to do in case of an emergency. Knowing CPR always makes people feel more secure and is a good qualification for any parent as well as for anyone who cares for children.

Who can watch my baby? Do I need to find special nursing care?

Mr. Sklenar: Again, this depends upon your baby's medical condition, something to discuss with a physician. In most cases, these children do not require any special nursing care, but need to be loved, fed, and played with like any other baby. A good childcare provider will feel comfortable with your baby's needs, have some experience in childcare, and have no physical or mental conditions that would hinder her performance.

How do I look for a caregiver?

Mr. Sklenar: You can find a caregiver through placement agencies; nanny-training programs; placing a classified ad; or referrals from relatives, friends, or coworkers. Your local National Association of Child Care Resource & Referral agency and national nanny organizations can inform you of placement agencies serving your area. Another option is to advertise in your local paper and on bulletin boards around your neighborhood. A caregiver is probably the most important employee you will ever hire, so set aside ample time to prepare for and conduct the interview(s) and to check references. Ask the candidate to provide you with names and phone numbers of previous employers.

"I changed jobs and childcare arrangements and was fortunate enough to find a close-by, flexible job and great childcare providers."

—*Laura Murphy, mom to Amanda*
(*hypertrophic cardiomyopathy and Noonan's syndrome*)

"She is currently taking seven different medications! My biggest fear was having to find a baby-sitter who could handle giving Alyssa the correct medications. Thank God we managed to find Lisa. Lisa is like Alyssa's second mom."

—Michelle Goenner, mom to Alyssa Mae
(dextrocardia, heterotaxy asplenic syndrome,
double outlet right ventricle, severe pulmonary stenosis)

CHAPTER 4
DAY-TO-DAY LIVING

Ruth Collins-Nakai, M.D., M.B.A.   Emily Jackness, M.D.
Amy R. DeFelice, M.D.   Wahida Karmally, M.S., R.D., C.D.E.
Arthur Garson, Jr., M.D., M.P.H.   Beth F. Printz, M.D., Ph.D.
William Gay, M.D.   Amnon Rosenthal, M.D.
Welton Gersony, M.D.   Dennis Sklenar, C.S.W.
                    Jonathan Slater, M.D.

Ah, the nitty-gritty. Not definitions of defects or specifics about surgical procedures, but the things you're likely to agonize over just as much if not more. Is your child eating enough, and if not, how can you make him eat more? How are you going to con your willful daughter into taking medicine, and what do you do if she spits it back out? When should you call your pediatrician and when should you call your cardiologist? Too hot? Too cold? Too much activity? Too little activity? We have worried about it all, and expect you have or will as well. This chapter includes enough medical answers and time-tested parental tricks and solutions to get you through a lot, but we bet you'll think of something we haven't and you'll be heading for the phone. And that's what you should do. Your child is your child, and if something doesn't seem right or if you're unsure about a situation, call and ask your doctor, even if it's in the middle of the night or just a day or an hour since the last time you called. That's what they're there for.

Gerri

Everyday Concerns

How can new parents tell if their baby has difficulty eating or shortness of breath?

Drs. Gersony, Printz, and Jackness: Sometimes it's difficult for a parent who doesn't have any experience in childcare. Obviously, the more serious the problem, the easier it will be to tell. If a newborn baby takes an hour to drink four ounces because he tires after every few sucks, this is evidence of difficult feeding. Regarding shortness of breath, you should call your doctor if your infant consistently breathes more than sixty times per minute. Also call your doctor if your baby pulls in his ribs or sternum (breastbone) while breathing fast, or if you think your baby is having difficulty eating or is experiencing shortness of breath.

What danger signs should I look for in my child after he's passed infancy?

Dr. Gay: Any time that you notice respiratory difficulty, especially if it's in any way unexplained, you should call your cardiologist. A change in the level of consciousness or passing out—we call it syncope—is another danger sign.

Tiredness may or may not be a danger sign—it depends on the type of tiredness you're seeing. If a child is tired, the vast majority of time it's not a heart problem. It's common, in fact, for adolescents to be tired. But if your child is tiring when he goes out to play with other kids, if he can't keep up and is short of breath, that's potentially bothersome. It's important for a doctor to pin down what you mean when you call and say "my child is tired."

My child has a murmur. Do I need to tell the school before he arrives?

Dr. Gay: If your child has had cardiac surgery or heart repair, or if surgery is planned for the future, then yes, the school should know. If your child has a functional murmur, I would not mention it to the school, as it's likely to cause unnecessary confusion or concern.

It's a good idea to ask your doctor how to handle the school. Your doctor can really help you, bearing in mind that you don't want your child treated differently in school if she doesn't need to be.

My child vomits several times a week. Could vomiting be associated with her heart defect?

Drs. Gersony, Printz, and Jackness: Babies who breathe very fast because of heart failure may have vomiting as one of their symptoms, although there are many other causes of vomiting in an infant or older child.

My baby sweats a lot. Could this be related to his heart condition?

Drs. Gersony, Printz, and Jackness: Many normal infants sweat, particularly when they are sleeping. On the other hand, infants and children with heart failure may also sweat with exertion (even if that exertion is merely eating or crying), just as adults sweat when they exercise.

My son looks a little blue after his bath. Should I be worried?

Dr. Garson: This is generally not a cause for concern. Many healthy infants have less blood going to their skin when they get cold, which makes their skin look a little bluish, often in the hands and feet or even around the mouth. This seems to be especially true in light-haired children.

Can my child get his routine childhood vaccinations?

Dr. Collins-Nakai: Absolutely! We encourage children with heart disease to have routine immunizations. We don't want them to be exposed to increased risk of polio or measles or whooping cough! The only exception to this is if your child has a compromised immune or defense system. Some children with heart disease also have problems with their immune system (e.g., children with DiGeorge syndrome). In those cases it is important to follow the advice of the immunologists and infectious-disease experts about which immunizations your child should receive.

Should my child get a flu shot?

Dr. Collins-Nakai: We encourage children with heart disease to have routine flu shots each year. The flu shots protect children against influenza virus infection, which can cause fever, muscle aches, headaches, and very bad chest infections or pneumonias. ("Flu" does not mean tummy upset— which medical people refer to as "gastro.")

Under what circumstances should I call my pediatric cardiologist immediately, and when should I wait until business hours to call?

Dr. Rosenthal: The occurrence of a blue (cyanotic) spell, fainting, sudden and unexpected shortness of breath, irregular or very rapid heart rate, and the onset of chest pain or severe back pain all warrant an immediate call to your pediatric cardiologist. Urgency depends on the symptoms or changes expected for specific heart defects as discussed with the cardiologist. In general, call your pediatric cardiologist during business hours if your child has symptoms such as edema (swelling around the eyes or the feet), an increase in the severity of the blueness or shortness of breath, brief palpitations, or fever of an unexplained nature that has lasted more than three to four days. Other, less urgent issues may include questions about cardiac medications or drug interaction, concerns about scheduled procedures, or precautions prior to noncardiac surgery. Changes in heart condition tend to occur more rapidly in newborns than older children, so parents of a newborn shouldn't hesitate to call the physician.

"If you call at a weird time and it turns out to be nothing, you have permission to be relieved and not feel guilty for calling."
— *Robin Yankow, mom to Eddie (aortic stenosis and enlarged aortic root)*

Can I trust my child's ability to limit herself, or do I need to set limits?

Dr. Gay: In younger children, you don't need to set limits except under really special circumstances, as dictated by your doctor. In older children, some conditions are serious enough that we don't want the children participating in competitive football, wrestling, weight lifting, etc.—sports that involve serious strenuous exertion. Your doctor should give you specific recommendations about physical activities.

Does stress affect my child's heart?

Dr. Rosenthal: Stressful situations are an integral part of life and clearly may also affect the response of the child with a heart problem. Occasionally emotions or stress may induce rhythm disturbances. Children who are known to have underlying heart muscle problems, insufficient blood flow or oxygen delivery to the heart, or certain electrical heart problems may be more prone to rhythm problems. For example, stress may induce ventricular tachycardia in children with prolonged QT syndrome, supraventricular tachycardia in those predisposed to fast atrial rhythm abnormalities, increased blueness in the cyanotic child, or chest pain in the youngster with cardiomyopathy or narrowing of the aortic valve. Stress is most likely to affect those with specific underlying heart conditions.

Does extreme temperature (hot/cold) affect my child's heart?

Dr. Rosenthal: The effect of exposure to extreme temperature, hot or cold, depends on the severity and duration of the exposure as well as the specific heart condition and whether the individual is resting or exercising. Cyanotic and/or polycythemic children (those with low blood oxygen and/or very thick blood) don't generally tolerate prolonged exposure to hot weather. They often require air conditioning and adequate fluid intake to prevent dehydration. Children with heart failure or poor circulation experience increased symptoms with prolonged exposure to hot weather because their heart may not be able to pump enough to increase blood flow adequately. Similarly, children with narrow valves or heart muscle stiffness may not tolerate extremes in temperature because of a decrease in venous blood return to the heart. Excessive sweating and water loss may further increase their symptoms. Exposure to cold, especially during exercise, may increase blood pressure and heart rate and thus make the heart work harder. If there is insufficient oxygen reaching the heart muscle or if the heart is already functioning poorly, such as in children with a narrow aortic valve or heart muscle weakness, chest pain may result.

What effect will secondhand smoke have on my child's defect? Is it more dangerous for him than for a healthy child?

Dr. Gay: Secondhand smoke isn't good for anyone, but it won't have any additional effect on the underlying abnormality of your child's heart. However, any time a child is prone to respiratory difficulties, especially if he's prone to wheezing or bronchial spasms, secondhand smoke can cause problems.

My daughter has tetralogy of Fallot, and my cardiologist told me not to let her cry. Why?

Drs. Gersony, Printz, and Jackness: Some children with tetralogy of Fallot (who have not yet had surgery) have episodes of increased cyanosis when they are agitated. They may have a reflex reaction whereby the flow of blood to their lungs continues to decrease, making them bluer and bluer until they can pass out. These episodes tend to occur in the morning, and are not necessarily associated with crying. An infant with tetralogy of Fallot in the care of a pediatric cardiologist is not necessarily prone to tetralogy spells, and crying will not cause symptoms. No parent can prevent an infant from crying on occasion.

Is the Ferber method (where parents are encouraged to let their child cry—sometimes for an extended amount of time—in the process of teaching them to fall asleep by themselves) safe for my child?

Drs. Gersony, Printz, and Jackness: As a general rule, it is acceptable to use the Ferber method, keeping in mind that other reasons for crying should be excluded. The one exception to using the Ferber method is if your child has tetralogy of Fallot, in which case you should discuss it with your doctor.

What can I do if I think my child is having a "tetralogy spell"?

Drs. Gersony, Printz, and Jackness: Most important is to comfort your child in your arms. You should put your baby's knees to his or her chest, which increases the amount of blood flowing to the lungs. If your baby continues to be agitated and blue, or if he or she doesn't respond normally, this is a medical emergency and you should call your pediatric cardiologist immediately or go to an emergency room. In any event, even if your child recovers immediately, you should report the episode to your physician.

Can I let my baby crawl?

Drs. Gersony, Printz, and Jackness: You do not need to restrict your baby's activity. Babies will restrict their own activity and not do any harm to themselves in this way.

My child needs to limit her physical activity. How do I accomplish this without drawing attention to her?

Mr. Sklenar: Children's work is to play and have fun. Your child may have to restrict how much energy she exerts during these activities, and you don't want her to feel differently than her peers or to feel left out of any activity. It is important to involve your child in activities that aren't as physically assertive, but yet rewarding and enjoyable to the child. Be positive about what your child can do rather than focus on what she cannot do. Work together to find activities that serve to build confidence and self-esteem. For example, if your child is unable to play on the baseball team, she may still participate by keeping score or assisting the coach. Encourage your child to explore special-interest clubs and classes that may provide a sense of inclusion as well as fun and learning. (See chapter 7 for more on limitations.)

"I find that my child does not like to be treated differently or have limitations placed on her."
>   —*Yolanda Scott, mom to Ondrea (dextocardia mitral atresia, pulmonary atresia, interrupted IVC, dual permanent pacemaker)*

Can my son be circumcised?

Drs. Gersony, Printz, and Jackness: Yes. There is no medical contraindication to circumcising a baby with heart disease, as long as the baby is not acutely ill. This, too, can be discussed with your doctor.

Should I get trained in CPR?

Drs. Gersony, Printz, and Jackness: There are very, very few children with heart disease who are at an increased risk for having an episode that would warrant CPR. However, it is always a good idea for parents and other caregivers to get CPR training, whether their children have heart disease or not.

What are some of the most common side effects children with CHD experience, and what are some of the most troublesome? Is there anything I can do to lessen or ease the side effects?

Dr. Collins-Nakai: Different types of heart disease cause different side effects. For instance, blue babies have low oxygen levels in their blood. We don't like to have those levels constantly below 70 percent because we know now from following many children for many years that if the levels are below 70 percent for long periods of time that the baby's development may not be normal. Therefore, for blue babies, your doctor will be measuring oxygen saturations at each visit. Other than seeing your doctor regularly and reporting when you think the baby is becoming more blue, there is nothing much you can do directly in these cases.

For children with heart failure, the problem is usually poor growth. Feeding these children small but very frequent meals is most helpful to keep them growing. All children with heart disease require some activity, so it is important to encourage all children to play normally. For some types of heart disease, your cardiologist will restrict your child from doing coached competitive sports. For the most part, some type of regular activity, such as walking, swimming, bike riding, or rollerblading, is recommended to keep them as fit as possible. Many children with heart disease will tire more quickly than normal, but that doesn't mean the child shouldn't be active! Just allow the child to stop when he or she is tired.

What is a normal heart rate?

Drs. Gersony, Printz, and Jackness: There is a very wide range of normal heart rates that varies with age and may range from 60 to 150 beats per minute while the child is resting comfortably. Babies' heart rates are greater than 100 beats per minute even while sleeping. Most important is that the heart rate responds appropriately to exercise (or increased activity), meaning that it increases gradually, and returns to normal soon after stopping.

What is a normal breathing rate? Is it okay if the rate drops when my child is sleeping?

Drs. Gersony, Printz, and Jackness: Again, there is a wide range of normal breathing rates for children. Newborn babies normally breathe twenty to forty times per minute. Many babies have "cyclical" respirations where they breathe rapidly for a few seconds, then slow down. This also is normal. A sustained respiratory rate of more than sixty per minute is considered high for newborns, but a rate of more than thirty per minute would be considered elevated for school-age children. It is perfectly normal for the respiratory rate to drop while a child is sleeping.

Could my baby have a heart attack?

Dr. Garson: Heart attacks in infants and children are extremely rare. A heart attack is almost always due to a blockage of one of the blood vessels actually nourishing the heart itself (coronary artery) and is caused in the majority of cases by a buildup of cholesterol on the inside of that artery. When the buildup is severe enough and a blood clot closes off that vessel, the heart muscle beyond the vessel may become injured or die. This is essentially a disease of adults, not of children. In the very rare event where a young child or an athlete dies suddenly, it is said to be due to a "heart attack," but this is very rarely the case.

Eating and Nutrition

Why do babies with heart failure have feeding problems?

Drs. Gersony, Printz, and Jackness: In the presence of a failing heart, the baby will almost always breathe fast. This is due to a "backup" or congestion in the lungs because the heart cannot move blood forward as effectively as in the normal state. When a baby is forced to breathe more frequently, it is difficult for him or her to feed. Eating or crying for a baby is really an "exercise stress test," where the heart has to increase how much blood it pumps to make up for increased demand. Furthermore, the work of breathing increases the caloric needs, and the infant's energy level is low. This combination of factors may lead to a failure to thrive. Virtually every form of heart disease that causes "congestive heart failure" should have vigorous medical and/or surgical treatment to avoid chronic feeding problems.

"I wanted to breast-feed him to help make him strong. I pumped as soon as he was born, till the day he was discharged. They wanted me to pump and feed him a bottle, because it was harder work for him to suck from the breast, but I found that to be very difficult. I put him to the breast and it was hard in the beginning, but he did great. He nursed constantly. I even used to nurse him while walking around with him in a sling, and I felt good that he was able to get the advantages of the breast milk."

—*Laura Ulaszek, mom to Brian (HLHS)*

Should I feed my baby more often or start her on solids earlier?

Drs. Gersony, Printz, and Jackness: Babies with heart failure often do better with small volume, frequent feedings. Instead of feeding every four hours, it is common for babies with heart failure to feed every two to three hours. This is equivalent to you taking frequent breaks when exercising at the gym rather than running a marathon. It is helpful to increase the caloric content in the babies' formula without increasing its volume. Breast milk and standard formulas normally supply twenty calories per ounce. Many formula producers supply "enhanced calorie" formulas, which may have as much as 50 percent more calories per ounce versus their standard formula. There are also ingredients that you can add to standard formula or pumped breast milk to increase its caloric content. (See "If Your Child Is Having Feeding Problems" later in this chapter.) By drinking such formulas, a baby can drink the same caloric content without having to drink as much volume. Starting a baby on solid foods earlier will not increase the supply nor decrease the demand these babies have, as solid foods actually contain less calories per ounce than breast milk or formula.

Is there anything else I can do to help her gain weight?

Drs. Gersony, Printz, and Jackness: Some pediatric cardiologists advocate placement of feeding tubes, either continuously or only at night, to increase the caloric (or energy) supply without the demand inherent in a baby actually drinking. Tube feeding is usually only needed in cases of severe heart failure. If at all possible, a baby's heart defect should be surgically corrected before the infant is malnourished and requires tube feeding.

If my child's growth has been following a steady curve, but is only at the 0–5th percentile for age, should I be increasing her calories?

Drs. Gersony, Printz, and Jackness: Steady growth (height, weight, and head circumference) along a curve is a sign that your child is most likely receiving adequate calories. Many factors influence which percentile a given child will follow, most important of which is usually the size and growth pattern of other family members.

My doctor told me that my child can eat anything, the more fattening, the better, but I'm doubtful this will really make him grow taller and bigger. I don't want to end up with a short, fat kid with bad eating habits.

Ms. Karmally: Your doctor wants your child to get sufficient calories for growth and development. These calories should come from "nutrient dense" foods. Rather than offering your child a doughnut (mainly hydrogenated fat and sugar!) for breakfast, give French toast prepared with milk and eggs and a topping of fruit. Even a slice of pizza for breakfast would be preferable to a doughnut! The pizza will provide protein and calcium from the cheese.

At the same time, don't label high-fat, high-sugar foods as "forbidden." All foods can be part of your child's healthy meals.

Get the child involved in meal preparation and food shopping. Even finicky eaters will be more likely to eat foods they help prepare.

Offer healthy foods with kid appeal. You can shape breads and cheese like their favorite cartoon characters; serve small pieces of fruit on bamboo sticks as "kabobs"; and serve frosty milk-fruit drinks or parfaits with toasted oats, yogurt, and berries.

When do eating habits form, and what can I do to instill good eating habits while still providing my child with the extra calories she needs?

Ms. Karmally: Your child learns to eat a variety of foods by watching your eating habits. It is important to eat with your child. Include a variety of healthy foods and give your child the freedom to choose and taste different foods in a relaxed and fun setting.

I've been told my child should be on a "heart-healthy" diet. What do you recommend?

Ms. Karmally: The typical American diet is linked with several health problems, including obesity, high blood pressure, elevated cholesterol levels, atherosclerosis, type 2 diabetes mellitus, and certain cancers. The typical American diet is high in fat (particularly saturated fat, which raises blood cholesterol levels), high in calories (causing weight problems and obesity), and low in fruits and vegetables.

Setting healthy eating patterns at an early age may be very helpful in preventing these problems later in life. If you are told that your child should be on a heart-healthy diet, your child should:

1. Eat a variety of foods to get all the essential nutrients because no single food has all the essential nutrients in the amounts needed.
2. Get sufficient calories for growth, development, and maintenance of body functions.
3. Include foods such as cereals; all varieties of grains such as wheat, rice, barley, quinoa, amaranth, oats, and millet; fruit; vegetables;

legumes; nonfat and low-fat dairy products and fish; poultry without skin; lean red meats; and eggs.

Here are some other things you should know:

• Fruits, vegetables, and grains contain no cholesterol and generally are low in fat (exceptions are avocados and olives). All animal or flesh foods contain cholesterol in varying amounts (an egg yolk has 213 mg of cholesterol; 3 oz of chicken without skin or red meat has approximately 75 mg of cholesterol; shellfish, squid, and organ meats are high in cholesterol). The recommendation is not to exceed 300 mg of cholesterol per day.

• Processed foods can be high in calories, fat, and sodium (salt). The "nutrition facts" label on food packages will list the grams of fat and saturated fat, milligrams of sodium and cholesterol, and calories. Foods prepared with tropical oils (coconut, palm, palm kernel, and cocoa butter) as well as hydrogenated shortening should be limited. These fats raise blood cholesterol.

• The ingredients on the label are listed in order of greatest amount; the first ingredient on the label is the one contained in the product in the greatest amount.

• Low-fat cooking methods such as baking, broiling, microwaving, and steaming are best. For sautéing and stir-frying, use cooking spray or small amounts of unsaturated oils such as canola or olive.

• Snacking is part of your child's eating pattern. Snacks could be low-fat milk puddings, fresh fruits, vegetables with low-fat yogurt, trail mix made with whole grain cereal, dried fruits (raisins, dates, apricots, etc.), or sliced nuts.

• Children's appetites change from day to day. There could be "high-fat days" and "healthier days." To assess your child's eating habits, look at what he or she eats over several days.

• Change eating and exercise habits gradually for meaningful results. The American Heart Association publishes a number of heart-healthy cookbooks, including one for kids.

Are there certain foods that should be avoided while breast-feeding because they might harm a baby with CHD?

Drs. Gersony, Printz, and Jackness: Most babies with congenital heart disease will not be affected by any food or drink that their breast-feeding mother may take in. However, if your baby has an arrhythmia (disorder of the heart's rhythm), you should discuss the mom's intake of caffeine and any medications, herbs, and supplements, including over-the-counter cold medications, with your doctor.

Does my child need a special low-fat or low-cholesterol diet?

Drs. Gersony, Printz, and Jackness: No, there is no need to give your child less fat or cholesterol than what's in a normal, heart-healthy diet (see pages 88–89). Some of the caloric supplements that are given to babies with heart failure actually add extra fat in the form of triglycerides. No children (with or without heart disease) up until age two years should be given reduced-fat milk products (i.e., skim, 1%, or 2% milk), as they need fat in their diet for normal development of their body and brain.

You must remember that congenital heart defects are not related to coronary arteriosclerosis (hardening of the arteries), and the low-cholesterol diet issue is not a specific consideration in an infant with a congenital heart defect.

Should my child get his cholesterol checked?

Drs. Gersony, Printz, and Jackness: Children with congenital heart disease are not thought to have an increased risk for coronary artery disease. Having said this, all children (especially those whose families have a history of coronary artery disease or stroke) should have a screening test to check their cholesterol by the time they are teenagers. There are families who have inheritable forms of high cholesterol or triglycerides unrelated to congenital heart disease, where children may benefit from early intervention (including diet, exercise, or even medication in rare cases). A cholesterol screening test involves drawing a small amount of blood (about a tablespoonful), often before breakfast.

Should I limit my child's salt intake?

Drs. Gersony, Printz, and Jackness: Only in very rare cases of severe heart failure caused by poor function of the cardiac muscle itself is it necessary to limit your child's salt intake. As with everything in life, however, moderation is the best policy. All children, regardless of the presence of heart disease, should be given a heart-healthy diet rich in fruits and vegetables, low in saturated fats, and without excess salt.

Does my child need iron supplements?

Dr. Collins-Nakai: Your doctor will tell you if your child needs iron supplements. Sometimes, after a procedure such as a cardiac catheterization or heart surgery where there has been some loss of blood, your doctor will prescribe iron supplements for a couple of months to help the body rebuild the blood (hemoglobin) level. For most children who eat a normal diet, iron supplements aren't necessary once they have started solid food.

If Your Child Is Having Feeding Problems

What are safe, healthy ways to increase an infant's calorie intake?

Ms. Karmally: The goal for infant feeding is to provide enough calories and nutrients to support a baby's growth and development. Both breast and bottle feeding with infant formula can provide the adequate nourishment. Babies may lose a little weight soon after birth; that's considered normal. If your baby does not regain the weight within two to three weeks, your doctor will assess your infant's nutrient consumption. You can monitor the number of wet diapers (six or more every twenty-four hours) to make sure your infant is getting enough to eat.

You can safely increase calories when your baby is four to six months (when an infant stops pushing food out of his or her mouth, can support his or her head, and can sit up with help), initially with an iron-fortified rice cereal and later a barley cereal. Strained baby fruits are appropriate at five to six months. When chewing motion begins, a baby can digest strained meats and egg yolk (at six to eight months). At eight to nine months, when chewing improves with the presence of teeth, try junior foods or mashed/chopped table foods such as meat, poultry, potato, and chopped canned fruit. When your baby has more ability to chew (ten to twelve months), offer casseroles with pasta, rice, and chopped meats. Always check with your pediatrician before starting solids. Some foods may produce allergic reactions in some children.

Dr. DeFelice: Here's what I might recommend. (Always consult your doctor first to ensure that you are adding these substances in safe quantities.)

- Concentrating formulas
- Adding cereal to formulas
- Adding a powder called Scandical that dissolves into the formula
- Adding polycose, which are glucose polymers
- Adding fats in moderation in the form of liquid emulsions

What if I'm breast-feeding? How do I add these substances?

Dr. DeFelice: Breast-feeding is a terrific way to nourish your child. But if your baby isn't getting the calories he or she needs, you may want to pump your breast milk for a while and feed it to your child from a bottle. This way you can not only measure how much your child is taking but also put additives such as formula powder in to boost the calories. We have even given breast milk through feeding tubes.

What are safe, healthy ways to increase a child's calorie intake once he is eating regular table foods?

Ms. Karmally: While toddlers grow at a slower rate than infants, toddlers need enough energy to fuel their activities and the next stages of growth. Healthy eating from the get-go helps to establish a foundation of good nutrition. Include a variety of foods: whole milk; soft cheeses; regular yogurt (low-fat milk and low-fat dairy products are not recommended for children under two years of age); meat; chicken; fish; eggs; smooth peanut butter; sweet potato; chopped fruits; cereal; bread; and pasta prepared with oils such as olive, canola, or corn in the meal plan. I also recommend vegetables. However, if your baby needs more calories, choose more caloric-healthy foods. Vegetables are relatively low in calories. Because of their small stomachs, children may need to eat several times a day (six to seven times). Offer nutritious snacks between meals.

If your child seems overweight, discuss your concerns with your pediatrician. Restricting calories can be harmful to young children because low-calorie diets will not supply the fuel and nutrients necessary to grow and develop both physically and mentally.

When should a child be given a feeding tube?

Dr. DeFelice: Each child is an individual. The average child needs 100 calories per kilo. A child with a heart defect who is having trouble eating and gaining weight should probably get between 130 and 150 calories per kilo. If the child is not gaining weight and growing after you have done everything to increase his or calories orally, then it's time to consider a feeding tube.

Describe the different types of tubes available and the advantages of each.

Dr. DeFelice: A feeding tube bypasses the mouth and esophagus so that getting nutrition is passive. This way the babies' hearts don't have to work hard for sucking and swallowing. There are several different types:

Nasogastric (NG): This tube passes through the nose with the tip ending in the stomach.
Oralgastric: This tube goes through the mouth and into the stomach. It is pretty rare.

Gastrostomy: A hole is made in the child's skin, and the tube goes directly into the stomach. The hole heals once the tube is removed.

Jejunostomy: Similar to the gastrostomy, this tube goes directly into the jejunum.

Gastrojejunostomy: Part of this tube is in the stomach; part goes lower down, into the jejunum.

Nasoduodenal: This tube is similar to a nasogatric tube, but it goes from the nose through the stomach and continues into the intestine. This is used when the child has problems with vomiting or reflux.

What benefits are there to a feeding tube? What dangers or disadvantages are there?

Dr. DeFelice: A feeding tube helps children get the calories they need to help them to gain weight and grow. This is important for all children with heart defects, but particularly when you are preparing a child for surgery. We even think that their postoperative recovery is easier if they are better nourished.

There also are some drawbacks to feeding tubes:

- If you don't place the tube properly you could get food in the lungs, which can lead to severe pneumonia.
- Larger volumes of food may give the baby reflux or cause him or her to vomit. There also is a chance of aspirating the food when the baby vomits.
- Long-term NG tubes may cause pressure changes in the Eustachian tubes and may cause an increase in ear infections.
- Long-term NG tubes may cause problems with swallowing if your child doesn't have the chance to swallow for an extended period of time. He or she may have difficulties getting that skill back.
- Long-term NG tubes may occasionally cause delayed speech.

How can I expect a feeding tube to affect my child's eating habits after the tube is removed?

Dr. DeFelice: Many children do have problems regaining their oral feeding skills when their tube is removed. If possible, try to give the child half of his or her feedings orally while the feeding tube is in. Then, when you are trying to remove the feeding tube, gradually increase the amount of oral feedings.

How do you recommend I ease the transition from feeding tube to no feeding tube?

Dr. DeFelice: Go gradually as the child tolerates it. Children who have been on the feeding tube for the short term (a few months) usually don't have problems coming off. It can be more difficult when the child has had the feeding tube in longer.

Do you have any advice for parents when they are considering feeding tubes?

Dr. DeFelice: I usually tell parents that feeding tubes sound scary, but don't be afraid if your doctor feels that your child needs it. It is so important to make sure that these children are properly nourished.

We can teach most parents in a few days how to place the tubes and change the pumps. And there are always backup and support available to you if you need them. Also remember that it's not permanent, just a very effective way to help your child get the calories he or she needs to stay healthy.

Childhood Illnesses

How do I know when to call the primary care physician and when to call the cardiologist?

Dr. Rosenthal: Primary care physicians, whether pediatricians or family practice physicians, share responsibility with the pediatric cardiologist for providing comprehensive medical care to children with congenital heart problems. Questions relating to primary and preventive care such as immunizations, feeding schedules, and the diagnosis and management of common childhood illnesses are best addressed by the primary care physician. Questions relating to the diagnosis, management, or prognosis of a specific heart condition are deferred to the pediatric cardiologist. Many issues can and should be addressed by either one or both. These include, for example, coordination of care with other specialists; referral to community resources; professional or parent support groups; vocational guidance; and the need for antibiotics to protect against endocarditis, an infection.

The following table provides a suggested list of whom to call. Close communication between pediatric cardiologists and primary care physicians is essential for optimal care of the child with a heart condition, especially when major management decisions are made. Primary care is often neglected in the child with serious heart disease or during hospitalizations, and you should make every effort to make sure the primary care physician is informed and involved. Perhaps most important is to call when in doubt and call the most accessible physician or the one with whom you are most comfortable. And don't forget parent support groups and the Internet, both rich sources of information and support. There will likely be times when you'd rather ask another parent.

CONCERNS BEST HANDLED BY PEDIATRICIAN/PRIMARY CARE PHYSICIAN, CARDIOLOGIST, OR BOTH

	Primary Care Physician	Cardiologist
Prognostic implications of specific diagnosis		+
Cardiac medication–related problems		+
Coordination of case with other specialists	+	+
Growth and development	+	
Immunizations	+	
Nutrition/feeding	+	
Endocarditis prophylaxis	+	+
Dental care	+	
Social/behavioral/community service and support	+	+
Common childhood infections	+	
Activity/sports recommendations	+	+
Screening of associated noncardiac abnormalities	+	
Vocational/genetic counseling	+	+
Adolescent/sexual/pubertal	+	
Travel recommendations		+
School-related issues	+	

"When she was a newborn, she never cried. As an infant, she grunted a lot. Especially during the newborn phase, every new thing she did made us call the doctor."

—Roberta Love, mom to Allison (ventricular inversion, double outlet left ventricle, rudimentary right ventricle, transposition of the great arteries, VSD)

"I have learned to call the doctors and/or take Erin in to see them even when they tell me it's 'normal'—I follow my instincts."

—*Tracy Adams, mom to Erin (PDA, DORV, TGA, ASD, multiple VSDs, PA, small left ventricle, and severe PS of the left branch)*

If my pediatrician is treating my child for a virus or a bacterial infection, should I call my cardiologist also?

Dr. Gay: If your child has a serious underlying defect, is anticipating surgery, or has recently been through surgery, you should call your cardiologist. Otherwise it's not necessary.

Do I need to take special precautions to avoid common colds and infections or special measures when treating them because my child has CHD?

Dr. Gay: If you have an infant or a young child with a serious cardiac problem—for example, a condition that hasn't been repaired yet, or a residual abnormality that can't be repaired—something as basic as a cold can have a great deal more effect on your child. In that case it makes sense to take special precautions. Your doctor might even advise keeping that child out of day care. Those cases are really the minority.

A lot of children don't need special precautions, and it's just as important to know who they are. Especially today, when there are likely to be two parents working outside the home, there are a lot of stresses of everyday life. So you should make adjustments in the care of your child if you need to, but if you don't need to, taking extra precautions is not appropriate and is likely to bring on more stress unnecessarily. What's most important is to develop a good trusting relationship with a doctor who's willing to treat your child's case individually.

Is my child in more danger from exposure to infectious disease than others?

Dr. Gay: This really depends on the type of CHD your child has. If your doctor has suggested that your child needs to take special precautions, then, yes, infectious disease probably is more dangerous for your child. It really depends on the defect. Children with volume overload lesions or congestive heart failure treated with medicines have hearts that need to pump more blood than normal. Included in this category are infants or children with dysfunctional or decreased hearts (such as single ventricles). These are the types of cases in which infections can have more serious implications.

In what ways might a common virus or bacterial infection become a serious problem for a child with CHD?

Dr. Gay: Respiratory infections, which are mostly viral, are one example. If a child has a serious underlying problem, especially one associated with increased pulmonary blood flow, his or her respiratory infection could lead to pneumonia, and if he or she gets pneumonia she might be sicker than another child with pneumonia who doesn't have a heart problem.

"My older children were four and two when Brian was born. It was hard to keep the germs away. Brian had rotavirus and RSV between his Norwood and his Glenn procedures."

—Laura Ulaszek, mom to Brian (HLHS)

What common viruses and bacterial infections need to be watched with special care? What should we be watching for?

Dr. Gay: Watch for signs of dehydration with viruses and infections that involve stomach irritation, vomiting, and diarrhea. But the more serious concerns are infections that affect the child's breathing, his or her airway or lungs, because the heart and lungs are interrelated.

Any bacterial infection is serious for any child (not just a child with a heart condition) and should be treated by antibiotics. The only way to know if you're dealing with a bacterial infection is to go to the doctor.

I know that strep throat can lead to rheumatic fever. Is this of special concern to CHD kids?

Dr. Gay: This is a common question, but no, rheumatic fever is a different disease, and susceptibility to it is not increased by CHD. Strep throat should be treated just like any other bacterial infection, with special care taken if your child's CHD is serious enough to warrant it.

I have heard of viruses attacking hearts. Is my child at higher risk for this? What about after his repair?

Dr. Gay: Before or after the repair, the answer is no. Myocarditis (an inflammation of the heart muscle) is a horrible disease, and one of the most feared, because there's no specific cure—no surgery, no medicine. Some people's immune systems are more likely to react in an abnormal way to some viruses. So what happens is the immune system recognizes the heart muscle as foreign and attacks the heart, ultimately causing permanent dysfunction of the heart. This condition is much less common than CHD and is in no way related to CHD.

Does my child need antibiotics every time she has an infection to protect her heart?

Dr. Collins-Nakai: Antibiotics work against bacterial infections. They do not work against viruses. Therefore, antibiotics are necessary when there is a chance that a bacterial infection will cause a blood infection that could go to the heart. Such circumstances include dental work, including dental cleaning (because the gums are disturbed, and the human mouth contains many bacteria that can cause infections); major surgery; or in older children or adults, insertion of an intrauterine device (type of contraceptive), or childbirth. Infections such as common colds or other obviously viral infections do *not* require antibiotics unless your child has had a fever continuously for more than thirty-six to forty-eight hours. (Most viruses cause fever for only twenty-four to thirty-six hours. However, if your child has a prolonged fever with a viral infection, it may mean he or she is developing a complication that does require antibiotics.)

In summary, on most occasions when children become ill, it's viral and they don't require antibiotics.

My baby has a cold. Can I give him over-the-counter medication?

Drs. Gersony, Printz, and Jackness: Most children with heart disease will not be harmed if given over-the-counter medication, unless your child has an arrhythmia. However, certain decongestants tend to speed the heart and never should be overused. If your child is on medication for a heart problem, you should discuss giving your child any other medication with your doctor. Always tell your doctor about any herbs or supplements you're considering for your child.

"As a parent of a child with CHD, we must carefully consider how each medication, even over-the-counter, will affect the heart functions of our child."

—*Laurie Beard, mom to Trevor*
(*tetralogy of Fallot, Down syndrome*)

Medications

My baby is on digoxin for her heart failure. What is that and how does it help her?

Dr. Collins-Nakai: Digoxin is a drug which has been used for centuries for the treatment of heart failure. It comes from the foxglove plant and it works in two ways:

1. It slows down the heart rate so that it allows the heart to fill properly and completely. When the heart rate is too fast, the heart doesn't have time to fill properly and then the heart doesn't pump enough blood out to the body.
2. It increases what is called the "force of contraction" of the heart. This means that it increases the strength of the squeeze as the heart pumps the blood out to the body.

Together, the two actions of digoxin improve the efficiency of the heartbeat. Studies in adults have shown that digoxin makes people with heart failure feel better, and people on digoxin have less likelihood of being readmitted to hospital. For infants, it appears that digoxin helps to give them more energy for eating and seems to help them be less tired.

What is a diuretic and how does it work?

Dr. Collins-Nakai: A diuretic is any substance which increases urine output—in other words, it makes a person pee! Different diuretics act in different ways. Most diuretics act on the kidney. The most common diuretic used in patients in heart failure is Lasix (brand name) or furosemide (no-name or generic brand). It acts in the kidney in various places, primarily on the Ascending Loop of Henle. It is therefore called a "loop" diuretic. It works by blocking water and salts (electrolytes) from getting back into the blood after they have been filtered by the kidney. It forces the body to lose excess water and electrolytes especially potassium, sodium, chloride, calcium and magnesium. It helps people in congestive heart failure by getting rid of puffiness in the body and extra water in the lungs.

Why don't I just restrict the amount of fluid my baby gets?

Dr. Collins-Nakai: If you restrict the amount of fluid your baby gets, you also restrict the number of calories he or she receives. If the baby doesn't get enough calories she won't grow. And it turns out that babies in heart failure require more calories than normal to grow, so they require, if anything, an increased amount of fluid and calories to keep on growing. The other problem with restricting the amount of fluid for the babies in heart failure is that there then is no way to replace the salts or electrolytes they lose, and they develop imbalances in the electrolytes in their blood which can cause additional problems with heart and brain function.

What is an ACE inhibitor? What is it used for?

Dr. Collins-Nakai: An ACE inhibitor is a class of drugs called an-giotensin converting enzyme inhibitors. The action is a little bit complex: angiotensin is a substance in the body which is present in two forms, angiotensin 1 and angiotensin 2. Angiotensin 1 is an inactive form and must be converted or changed to angiotensin 2, the active form of the substance.

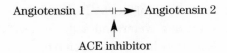

The substance which triggers the change from form 1 to form 2 is called angiotensin converting enzyme. Angiotensin 2 causes vessels to constrict or become smaller. When vessels leaving the heart constrict, two things happen: the blood pressure goes up, and the heart has to push harder to get the blood out to the body. The measurement which is used to quantify the amount of "push" needed to get blood out to the body is called peripheral arterial resistance or systemic vascular resistance. An ACE inhibitor blocks the change of angiotensin 1 to angiotensin 2.

Angiotensin 1 ⟶⊣⟶ Angiotensin 2
⬆
ACE inhibitor

There is less constriction of the arterial vessels, and sometimes, lower blood pressure. Therefore, the heart has to work less hard to pump the blood. ACE inhibitors are used primarily to lower blood pressure or to help the heart rest if the heart muscle is not working well. They are also used when valves in the heart are leaking a great deal as they allow the heart to push the blood out to the body at lower pressures so that there is not so much back pressure on the leaky valve. Different ACE inhibitors have different major effects and different side effects so that some are used in one situation whereas other types might be used for a different condition.

Why does my child need blood tests after taking her ACE inhibitor?

Dr. Collins-Nakai: All drugs have some side effects. One of the side effects which may occur is that ACE inhibitors may cause the white blood cell count in the blood to be low, or the potassium level in the blood to be higher than normal. They may also cause protein loss in the urine. Therefore, after an ACE inhibitor has been started, and usually once or twice a year thereafter, your doctor will want to check the blood and urine to make sure that everything is normal.

What is a beta blocker? What is it used for?

Dr. Collins-Nakai: A beta blocker is a class of drug which blocks the effects of catecholamines in the body. Catecholamines are the stress substances that cause your heart to pound when you are frightened. There are receptors or "parking places" for catecholamines in various tissues of the body, especially in the heart and lungs. When these substances can't get at the heart tissue because they have been "blocked," it causes the heart to slow down, and may cause the blood pressure to fall. Beta blockers are used to treat rapid heart rhythm problems, to treat high blood pressure (hypertension), and in recent years they have been used in patients with heart failure, as it has been shown that these people feel better and survive better if they take beta blockers. They are also used in people who have had a heart attack, and for people with delicate vessel walls (such as Marfan's syndrome). Again, there are many types of beta blockers, each with its own profile of major effects and side effects. Your doctor may use one type of beta blocker for one situation and another type to treat something else.

The current recommendations for patients with congestive heart failure is that they should receive all four classes of drugs together in order to obtain the best outcome: digoxin, diuretics, ACE inhibitors and beta blockers. This is considered now to be "maximal medical therapy" for heart failure.

What is the advantage to keeping my baby on medicine—why not repair his heart as soon as possible?

Dr. Collins-Nakai: When it is possible to repair your baby's heart immediately, this will be done. Sometimes it is better to allow the baby to grow a little before repair, and sometimes, it is necessary to wait until the pressure in the lungs drops enough, or until the vessels grow a little. The decision to operate is always a balance of what is best for the baby, what will give the best outcome, and what is the risk of operating at that time. We never want to operate until it is necessary, but we also don't want to stall and end up with problems from not operating sooner. Your cardiologist and cardiac surgeon will discuss these risks and benefits with you, and help your family to decide whether it is better to stay on medicines for a while and allow the baby to grow, or whether it is best to operate immediately.

If my child is doing well on medicine, what is the point to having open-heart surgery. Why can't he just stay on medicines?

Dr. Collins-Nakai: The medicines don't normally "fix" congenital heart disease. This type of disease does not mean that the heart muscle is sick and doesn't function. What it means is that the structure is not normal. It is like having a house built with the doors and windows in the wrong place. Only reconstructing the house will fix it. Similarly, with your child's heart, if there is a hole in the heart or a valve is too small, the medicines will help your child's heart cope with the extra load while the child is growing, but will not solve the underlying problem. Even if the child seems to be OK on the medicines, if there is a structural problem, eventually it will have to be fixed. Sometimes, with time, if the problem is not fixed, it can result in lung damage or kidney damage or other problems in adulthood. Your doctor will discuss with you the best time to have a low risk for the surgery, but a high benefit for your child.

I missed a dose of my child's medicine. How important is this? Should I double the dose next time?

Dr. Collins-Nakai: If you recognize that you missed your child's medicine within one to two hours after the dose was due, you can give the medicine at that time, and then just resume your normal medicine schedule. However, if it is longer than one to two hours, forget that missed dose, and just proceed to the next dose at the next time. Sometimes in very sick patients, drugs must be given at exact times, but these patients are usually in the hospital and watched carefully by nurses. For patients at home, one missed dose is not a problem, so long as it is only ONE missed dose. Do NOT double the dose the next time, as each drug is given in a dose that is appropriate for the weight of the child and doubling the dose may cause problems.

Do I need to give the medicine with meals?

Dr. Collins-Nakai: Your doctor or pharmacist will tell you whether or not you must give a particular medicine with meals. Many medicines may be taken with meals, but there are some medicines that must not be taken with meals as food interferes with the way the medicines are absorbed by the stomach.

My child is refusing to take his medication. How can I encourage him?

Dr. Collins-Nakai: Most children will learn to take medicine easily if it just becomes a routine. For infants, the medicines will be liquids, and the trick is to put the dropper into the side of the mouth but very far back and squirt the medicine into the back of the mouth so the baby has no choice but to swallow it. For older children, when you are teaching them to swallow pills, place the pill in the center of the tongue and as far back as possible, then give them a drink of a favorite juice or milk. Praise them when they do it well and it soon becomes routine. Sometimes it is necessary to grind up a pill and put it in applesauce or yogurt on a spoon (again far back in the mouth).

Some medicines taste terrible! For instance, a liquid that is often used to sedate children for procedures, called chloral hydrate, tastes quite bitter and almost mentholated. Again the trick is to get the medicine far back in the mouth so they are forced to swallow, followed by something they like (liquid or solid).

Dr. Slater: You may not be able to persuade him. Children generally hate to take medicine, especially if it is several times a day, and if it tastes foul. Try to make it fast, wash it down fast with something that tastes good, and don't have extended discussions and battles about it. Give him some limited choices about it to help him have some sense of control (i.e. over the timing, what they wash it down with, what fun thing they want to do after they're done, where in the kitchen or bathroom they want to be when they swallow it), but be clear that there is no choice about taking the medicine. Be firm but not angry about it, it just has to happen, and the faster this is accepted, the faster it can happen. Positive reinforcement such as stickers can sometimes work in younger children, when accompanied by a more systematic behavioral modification system. Most importantly, if you are having terrible battles over medication administration, get professional help; there are developmental pediatricians, psychiatrists and psychologists with specific training to assist with this.

TIPS FOR GIVING MEDICATIONS

"We didn't want to hide it in food, because philosophically we wanted him to know he was taking medication, because this is something he will need to do for his whole life."
—*Robin Yankow, mom to Eddie (aortic stenosis with an enlarged aortic root)*

"I give the meds in the side of the cheek while my son is taking a bottle . . . Never do I mix the meds in the bottle because it changes the taste of the formula and if my child refuses to finish the milk he does not get the meds."
—*Laurie Beard, mom to Trevor (tetralogy of Fallot, Down syndrome)*

"I pretend to feed it to her Pooh bear or another animal first, then give it to her."

—Tracy Adams, mom to Erin (PDA, DORV, TGA, ASD, multiple VSDs, PA, small left ventricle and severe PS of the left branch)

"We would mix all the morning meds or all the evening meds in one small bottle that the hospital gave us with a little bit of milk."

—Michelle Goenner, mom to Alyssa Mae (dextrocardia, heterotaxy asplenic syndrome, double outlet right ventricle, severe pulmonary stenosis)

"My daughter is nine months old so we put her medicine in about two ounces of liquid and feed her that when she gets hungry, before she gets any other food."

—Susan Wirth, nurse and mom to Julia (interupted aortic arch, VSD, ASD)

"My favorite trick for giving her medicine is the 'Medibottle' available through the 'Right Start' catalogue, and at certain discount stores. It ended our initial problems of having most of the medicine dribble out of her mouth."

—Alexandra Kraemer, mom to Cydney (transposition of the great vessels)

"As an infant, I dissolved her medication in warm water in an oral syringe and squirted it through the nipple of her bottle during feedings. Later, I squirted it directly into her mouth, then graduated to putting the pill in a spoonful of yogurt and now inside a Cheerio."

—Laura Murphy, mom to Amanda (hypertrophic cardiomyopathy and Noonan's Syndrome)

"I used plastic syringes and as soon as he was able to hold the syringe, I let him help give the med. If they are involved, you are not giving it to them, they are doing it themselves and they take the meds better. Praise, praise, praise for doing good!!"

—Sue Dove, mom to Scott (single ventricle)

"As an infant, we have found that holding his pacifier just slightly in his mouth allowed us to sneak the syringe in the corner of his now opened mouth. We would then squirt a little of the medicine in at a time. After each squirt, we would place the pacifier in his mouth and he would swallow the medicine as he sucked on the pacifier."

—Randy Sittner, dad to Isaiah (hypoplastic right ventricle, pulmonary atresia and tricuspid atresia)

"If we knew for sure that she didn't swallow it (the medicine), we would blow in her face and that would cause her to swallow the meds."

—*Deanna Lopez, mom to Christina*
(*pulmonary atresia stenosis, pacemaker*)

"Give medication through the nipple of a bottle. Remove the nipple from the bottle and place medication into nipple. Then give child nipple. Child will automatically suck."

—*Jackie Breckenridge and Calvin Bruton, parents to Tatiana*
(*AV canal, ostium primium ASD, inflow VSD,*
cleft and deformity of mitral and tricuspid valves)

"He takes medicines pretty well, but tends to spit out some if he is in an upright position, so it's best if he's slightly reclined."

—*Arlene Platten, mom to Joseph (AV canal and conjoined mitral valve)*

Are there other ways to give the medicine besides orally?

Dr. Collins-Nakai: Medicines can also be given through the veins (parenterally), through the skin, into the muscle or through the rectum. If the drug is being given intravenously, the child is usually in the hospital, so you won't have to worry about that at home. We try to avoid the intramuscular route in children (except for immunizations), and usually the only time the rectal route is used is if the child is vomiting a great deal and can't keep a medicine in the stomach.

Are there dangers if my child takes too much medicine?

Dr. Collins-Nakai: All medicines have side effects, and too much of one medicine may "poison" one or more of the systems in the body. Also some medicines interact with other medicines. So it is very important for your doctor to know all medicines that you are giving your child, including alternative, complementary or herbal therapies.

If there are problems with your child's liver or kidney function, the doses of medicines may have to be adjusted so that the levels in the blood are in the proper range for treatment.

Sometimes my child spits some of the medicine out or throws up afterwards. Should I give him more? How exact does the dosing need to be?

Dr. Collins-Nakai: If your child spits up or vomits the medicine within 5 to 10 minutes of you giving it to him or her, you may repeat the dose giving exactly the same amount. It is very common for babies to spit up especially when they have a cold. Often, the first regurgitation or spit-up contains a lot of thick mucous, which makes the baby feel sick and does not allow them to absorb their food or medicine. In that case, once the mucous is out of the tummy, the medicine and food will stay down.

If your baby spits up or vomits more than 10 minutes after you have given the dose, the baby may have already absorbed some of the dose. Therefore do NOT repeat the dose. Instead, wait until the time of the next dose, and give the normal dose at the next regular time. Do NOT double the dose the next time.

Just carry on with the regular medicine schedule. However, if your baby is vomiting continuously and has missed more than one dose of medicine because of vomiting, contact your doctor as the medicine may have to be given by another route (through an intravenous or IV). This sometimes happens when the baby or the child has an infection in the tummy called "gastro" (which is short for gastroenteritis, which means nausea and vomiting and/or diarrhea).

"I look at other mothers and I wonder what it would be like to just worry about the silly things."

—*Pam Rogers, mom to Hannah (AV canal)*

CHAPTER 5

SURGERY

Kathleen Grima, M.D.

Hillel Laks, M.D.

Larry Latson, M.D.

Martin O'Laughlin, M.D.

Dennis Sklenar, C.S.W.

Ross Ungerleider, M.D.

W E always knew that open-heart surgery was an eventuality for Lissie. Our original target was to wait until she was six months old before doing the surgery—assuming she didn't have any tetralogy spells or severe heart failure. As the months went by, she was doing so well that we decided we would wait longer to give her as much time as was possible to get big and strong. When she was a year old, we scheduled the surgery electively (a strange word when, believe me, the surgery was not my choice) for two months later.

In the weeks leading to the surgery, I promised myself I would be strong. I could see things rationally—we had one of the world's best surgeons at one of the world's best hospitals. It was, compared to many of the surgeon's cases, a very simple procedure. And this one surgery would fix the problem—after this Lissie would lead an active, healthy life and visit the cardiologist just once a year. With all this in mind, I vowed to be calm and upbeat, so as not to scare Lissie as we entered this strange environment.

That morning we waited in the anesthesia waiting room for our turn. Lissie played with the toys as Mat and I put on gowns so we would be sterile when we entered the operating room. As hard as this was for me, it had to be even harder for Mat. As a doctor and future cardiologist, he knew far too many negative possibilities.

They called our names and we scooped up Lissie and walked together into the brightly lit operating room. I looked around at the doctors and nurses all preparing the stage for our little girl. Before the surgery, I'd planned to make sure that the blood in the pump was the right type. I had heard horror stories of people dying from receiving the wrong type of blood, and this seemed like the one thing I could actually control in this very helpless situation. But when I went to ask, I found I couldn't speak, as I had already begun to cry. I held Lissie as the anesthesiologist put the mask on her face and guided her out of my arms. Mat took my hand, and we walked out the door. He held me and I sobbed for a while, then together we went upstairs to the waiting room.

Lissie came through the surgery with flying colors. Just a few days later she was running around the hospital, and less than a week after the surgery we were home. Many of the children who are diagnosed with CHD will need some form of surgery. Some surgeries will need to be performed within days of birth, others not for weeks, months, or even years. Some children are completely repaired in one operation, others will endure several over the course of their lifetime.

Many parents find it helpful to learn as much as possible about their child's surgery and/or catheterization. Ask your doctor about every possible treatment. Each surgeon may have a different approach to repairing a defect. This is especially true with hypoplastic left heart syndrome, where some doctors are in favor of the staged repair surgeries and others encourage transplant.

Whatever your child's diagnosis, you shouldn't be afraid to ask any questions you want. You'll feel a lot better during your child's surgery if you're informed about the procedure and confident in your decision. Remember—you are your child's best advocate.

Shari

Preop Questions and Concerns

While looking for a surgeon, I have heard the term "accredited program." What does this mean? How important is it?

Dr. Laks: In an "accredited program," medical specialists are board-certified if they have passed exams in an accredited program by the American Board of Medical Specialties, or board-eligible if they are in the process of taking exams. Surgeons must undergo recertification periodically to maintain their status with the board. Many, but not all, surgeons are also members of the American College of Surgeons, which recognizes the achievement of a surgeon who has successfully completed certification. A board-certified specialist has more experience and education than one who has not completed an accredited program.

Are there a minimum number of procedures a surgeon should do before operating on my child?

Dr. Laks: The American Board of Thoracic Surgery governs the training of heart surgeons. A surgeon must participate in a minimum number of procedures prior to being eligible for the examination for the American Board of Thoracic Surgery. A qualified surgeon would have completed training first in general surgery and then in cardiothoracic surgery. Once the surgeon has submitted a catalog of the procedures that he or she has performed or participated in as a first assistant in an accredited program, the surgeon becomes eligible for the examination process. Recertification ensures that the surgeon has performed the minimum number of cases during his or her career at the level the board considers acceptable.

One should also consider that certain defects are so rare that most surgeons won't have as much experience with them as with other defects. When choosing an institution or a surgeon for the treatment of congenital heart disease, ask how many of a particular defect the institution treats each year and what the outcomes are with regard to survival and complication rates. Normally this would be discussed during the informed-consent process. It's important to remember that published results of one institution may not necessarily be reproducible by another surgeon or institution.

How can I be sure that I am being told all of the treatment options? If my medical center does not offer me options in treatment, how can I find one that will?

Dr. Laks: Physicians are obligated to present all treatment options for a given diagnosis. This information must be discussed prior to agreement between the surgeon and the patient. The patient's cardiologist and surgeon would normally discuss this during the preoperative evaluation. Such discussions generally address the timing of surgery.

"When we finally scheduled Alexandra for surgery, we wanted to meet the surgeon. They gave us a hard time because his schedule was so busy. But it was important to us to meet the man who was going to be operating on our child, regardless of his incredible reputation. Don't be intimidated—if you want to meet them, do. Be your child's advocate."

—Pat Posada Klapper, mom to Alexandra (VSD)

When should I get a second opinion?

Dr. Laks: When considering a surgical option for the treatment of a congenital heart defect, a second opinion allows parents to see their child's symptoms in relation to the natural history of that defect. For example, there are instances in which surgery may be recommended for a child who essentially has no symptoms. This is because the natural history of the disease is well known and early intervention may be indicated. There are other instances when the complexity of the defect dictates two possible surgical treatments, depending on the "school of thought." In this situation, you should obtain a second opinion to ensure a more complete understanding of the controversies involved in the treatment of your child.

Consider a second opinion when "circulatory arrest" is contemplated as part of an operation. Certain procedures require that the body be drained of all its blood for the surgeon to reconstruct defective structures. This means there is no circulation of blood for a short time. The body is protected by cooling it down to levels at which the brain and the other organs are "turned off." This technique has been available since the 1960s, and some cooling (hypothermia, but not circulatory arrest) is routine for most open-heart surgery as a safety measure. Circulatory arrest is relatively safe for about forty minutes, and with current advanced techniques this time can be slightly extended. In general, since long-term effects on the brain are not completely known, it is always better to avoid circulatory arrest unless there is no other choice. Some defects (e.g., ventricular septal defect and aortic coarctation) can be repaired in two operations without circulatory arrest rather than one with circulatory arrest. Consider these options when you're planning elective surgery—weigh the advantages of each approach against the risks and experience of the surgeon.

Are certain procedures done at certain institutions, or do they do every type of procedure everywhere?

Dr. Laks: Large centers generally perform most or all of the cardiac surgical procedures. Smaller institutions without the infrastructure to support the highly complex procedures may refer these cases to a larger institution with concentrated experience. For example, an institution that performs a hundred pediatric cardiac surgical procedures per year would not have the same experience with complex reconstructions when compared to an institution that performs four hundred pediatric cardiac surgical procedures per year. There are many instances when a younger surgeon would ask an older, more experienced senior surgeon to assist during a complex surgical procedure. This ensures an additional level of safety for the operation.

"Find out from many different sources what is the best hospital and who is the best doctor for what your child has. Insist on going where you want to go. Don't let your insurance company tell you where to go if you have that option."

—*Anne Linne, mom to Kevin (transposition of the great vessels)*

"After he was born, Zachary was transferred to another hospital for surgery while I stayed at the hospital where he was born. My husband felt split, wanting to be at both hospitals, but I told him to be with Zachary. I had a friend come and stay with me for moral support. I felt myself detaching from the situation because Zachary was at the other hospital. I couldn't even pick up the phone to call the nursery to see how he was doing. Finally, on the day of his surgery, my OB insisted that I go over to the other hospital to see him. I probably checked out of the hospital before I should have, but I needed to be there."

—*Carole Stoll, mom to Zachary*
(VSD, subaortic stenosis, interrupted aortic arch)

What are the advantages of seeking surgical care near home, and when does it make sense to consider treatment farther away?

Dr. Laks: Pediatric cardiac surgery is generally available in most large cities in the country. There are smaller cities where pediatric cardiac surgery is performed less frequently and only on an urgent basis for the most simple operations. An important question to ask is: How experienced is the center performing the surgery? As the complexity of the diagnosis increases, the experience is more concentrated at the larger centers, and it's reasonable to consider treatment farther away from home.

I have heard that a certain hospital specializes in my child's defect. How do I get in touch with it?

Dr. Laks: Most major hospitals have single access numbers that are used to streamline inquiries to a specific specialty service. Parents may consult their pediatrician or pediatric cardiologist for this information. Since pediatric cardiology is a highly specialized field, most cardiologists know the location of specialized centers.

How do I know when it's time for my child to have surgery?

Dr. Laks: Timing of the surgery in the case of pediatric congenital heart defects is an important question. There are circumstances when surgery would be proposed even if the child has no symptoms. This is because the natural history of heart defects has been extensively documented in the past forty years, and it is often important to intervene before damage from the defect can occur. Generally speaking, nature has given the heart (and body) a large reserve of strength and energy to overcome many ailments. This reserve will diminish as the child grows and as the demand on a defective heart increases. There are other instances when surgery is required urgently because the child has severe symptoms. During the past fifteen to twenty years the trend has been to offer surgery to children at a younger age to prevent long-term damage to the heart from the defect. There are many centers that now treat newborns. Always question the indications for surgery at a very young age and ask what would happen if surgery were delayed for six months or for several years. There are other defects in which surgery isn't necessarily indicated for the newborn and may be timed more electively prior to the beginning of the school years.

My child seems to be doing okay, so why not put off the surgery as long as possible?

Dr. Laks: Putting off surgery as long as possible was once the treatment of choice in cardiac surgery. However, as surgery for congenital heart defects has become safer and as we've learned more about the natural history of congenital heart defects, we've reconsidered the timing of surgery. Often the pediatric cardiologist will observe the child at two or three intervals to see if the defect is causing any harm, even if the child has no symptoms. However, surgery may be indicated even without symptoms in situations where once they occur it may be too late to perform a successful surgical procedure. For example, in the case of one of the most common diagnoses, ventricular septal defect, surgery may be indicated prior to the end of the first year of life to prevent the occurrence of high blood pressure in the circulation of the lungs. Once this high blood pressure occurs, it would be too late to fix the defect, and there could be damage in the circulation to the lungs, which would then create a higher-risk situation.

What is the best age to do surgery?

Dr. Laks: Newborn children are very small, and certain organ systems, such as the kidneys, may not be completely mature. Surgery in the first three months of life is performed only if absolutely necessary. After the first three months of life, surgery is usually considered safer. Many defects are fixed in the first year prior to the time when the effect of the normal physiology may be irreversible. In the case of certain defects, the complexity of the surgery dictates that it would be easier to perform the operation when the child has grown and when the structures within the heart are easier to access and manipulate. Such children often have staged procedures over a number of years. In yet another situation, such as the one for atrial septal defects, surgery may be performed electively at any time during childhood, and in this situation parents often choose to get it done before the beginning of the school year to minimize any interruption in the normal progress of activities.

"Last time, 1996, we waited [to schedule surgery] until after Johnny had attended the All-Star baseball game—a great decision, wonderful memories."
—*Sandra Gravel, mom to Johnny*
(aortic stenosis, subaortic stenosis, coarctation)

[We scheduled surgery] during summer vacation, to have plenty of time to recuperate."
—*Deanna Lopez, mom to Christina*
(pulmonary atresia stenosis, pacemaker)

"Her second surgery was elective, sort of (homograft pulmonary valve placement), so I listened to advice from her pediatric cardiologist and the surgeon who recommended it. Then I did some research on my own and came to the conclusion to get it done now while she was healthy, rather than wait until something (her right ventricle) was failing."
—*Diane Barilko, mom to Alexandra (double outlet right ventricle,*
pulmonary atresia with a VSD, discontinuous LPA,
major aorto/pulmonary collateral arterials, pulmonary branch stenosis)

Is there a minimum age or weight for surgery?

Dr. Laks: There is no minimum age or weight for surgery. However, newborn babies with low birthweight are more delicate, and the risk of the operation must be weighed against the benefits. If there is no choice, the best compromise may be an intermediate procedure (less complex and not necessarily an "open" heart operation), followed, after a time, by a fully corrective operation. As the child grows and tissues mature, the second surgery becomes less risky.

Dr. Ungerleider: It is possible to place infants as small as 1 kg (2 lbs) on cardiopulmonary bypass (the heart/lung machine) and to attempt repair of their heart defect. It is distinctly unusual for babies who require heart surgery to be born this tiny. Nevertheless, heart surgery on infants who weigh less than 2 kgs is extremely challenging for the entire team (anesthesia, perfusion, surgery), and for this reason it is typical that extremely tiny infants are managed "medically" until they grow. Surgery would usually be offered only for those tiny infants who are in critical condition or who are not growing because of their heart defect.

What if my child gets sick before surgery? How sick does he need to be for the surgery to be delayed? Why can't you do the surgery if he's sick?

Dr. Laks: When a child is to undergo elective surgery, it's important for the child to be in optimal physical condition to tolerate the surgery. If a child has a cold, the lungs may be weakened and the stress of surgery may turn a simple cold into a significant pneumonia that could cause prolonged respiratory failure during the postoperative period. This may occur because open-heart surgery involves use of machines that divert the circulation outside of the child's body to maintain the child's brain and other organs while the surgeon operates on the heart and lungs. Although this is relatively safe, it is an unnatural route for the blood to pass through and therefore has certain effects that are termed "the inflammatory response." This response affects virtually every organ in the body and temporarily causes some dysfunction. Most healthy children and adults overcome this inflammatory response, which subsides after a few days. The ability to overcome the inflammatory response is greatly enhanced by the improvement of the heart following the operation.

"The second surgery was delayed because of illness. Nicholas had a pretty bad cold right before surgery. They had us put it off two weeks. I was very upset, because I had really psyched myself up for this. I knew it was too dangerous to put him through surgery with a cold, though. I wish I would have realized that it was no threat to Nicholas to put his surgery off a couple of weeks. It was really not a big deal to wait."

—*Deanna Smith, mom to Nicholas (HLHS)*

"Kevin's surgery was scheduled for the Friday after he was born. The surgeon was very tired that week and decided to postpone the surgery until Monday. I was devastated at the news. I was a wreck and didn't know if I could survive another weekend of waiting. The nurse explained that I would not want a tired surgeon performing surgery, which I understood. But it was still very tough on us."

—*Anne Linne, mom to Kevin (transposition of the great vessels)*

Blood Donations

Will my child receive blood or blood products during surgery?

Dr. Grima: Most babies will need at least one unit of blood to fill the cardiopulmonary bypass pump. Further blood usage depends upon the complexity of the surgery, and the number of units required will vary. The pediatric surgeon is the best source of information about blood requirements.

Should I bank blood? Is this safer than using the blood bank?

Dr. Grima: Blood is safer than ever. There is usually ample available blood to support these procedures. One's own blood (i.e., autologous blood) is the safest blood to get, but that is obviously not an option for infants. Directed donor blood has not been found to be safer than blood donated by the community, but often families feel uncertain about the safety of the blood supply and are uncomfortable if they don't provide blood themselves.

Is it possible to donate blood while I'm pregnant?

Dr. Grima: Pregnant women can only donate blood for themselves. Once the pregnant woman has delivered, she must wait six weeks before donating blood.

How soon before surgery should I give blood?

Dr. Grima: It depends on the age of the patient and the policies of the hospital's transfusion service and the surgeon. For newborns, some transfusion services use only blood that is fewer than five days old. In other hospitals, fresh whole blood twenty-four to forty-eight hours old is reserved for pediatric cardiac surgery. In still other transfusion services, a single unit is reserved for an individual infant and used for the shelf life of that unit, which is twenty-nine to forty-two days. In general, blood should be donated in time for the testing to be performed and the unit shipped to the hospital blood bank. The blood donation center should be helpful in advising donors of the appropriate time frame so that blood is tested, shipped, and fresh enough to be used for a particular patient.

Do donors have to be relatives?

Dr. Grima: Directed donors do not have to be relatives, and in fact blood donations from relatives have to be irradiated to prevent a rare complication of transfusion known as graft versus host disease, which shortens the shelf life of those units to four weeks. Directed donor units from individuals not related to the recipient generally are not irradiated, but this can vary depending on the policies of the collection center and the hospital.

What are the risks of getting AIDS or hepatitis from banked blood?

Dr. Grima: The risk of AIDS or hepatitis from banked blood is the same whether the blood comes from a community donor or a directed donor. For HIV, the risk from a single transfusion is estimated to be 1 in 676,000. For hepatitis C, the risk is 1 in 100,000 and for hepatitis B, the risk is 1 in 66,000. Directed donors differ from community blood donors in that they are often first-time donors and have not been previously tested for all the required viral markers. It is important that directed donors are true volunteer donors and do not donate because of pressure from relatives.

Newer tests are being developed that will further decrease the risk of transmitting these viruses. DNA testing, or NAT (nucleic acid testing), is being performed for HCV and HIV. This is a very sensitive test for these viruses but it is currently not a licensed test and is considered experimental. The risk of acquiring HCV from blood tested with this new assay is about 1 in 285,000 and is approaching 1 in 300,000. For HIV, the risk is less than 1 in a million. About 95 percent of the blood collected in this country is tested by this method.

Is there a charge to bank blood?

Dr. Grima: Donating for a particular individual adds to the processing cost for that unit of blood. The blood collection center must track the particular unit through donation, testing, and shipping so it arrives on time for the surgery. Blood centers either charge the donors for the additional costs of drawing these units or pass the costs on to the hospitals. However the costs are recovered, directed donation does add to the already high cost of blood products.

Do I need to be the same blood type as my child to donate blood?

Dr. Grima: For infants, type O blood is generally transfused. An O donor is the universal donor—all other blood types can receive type O. If the surgeon requests fresh, whole blood, then the blood type of the donor must be identical to the infant's. An infant who is Rh-positive can receive either Rh-positive or negative blood. Rh-negative infants can receive only Rh-negative blood.

In the Operating Room

What is cardiopulmonary bypass? Is it used in all surgeries? What are the possible complications from it?

Dr. Ungerleider: Cardiopulmonary bypass (CPB) is another name for the heart/lung machine. CPB was first used to perform open-heart surgery in 1953, but early machines were "primitive," and the technology was unreliable. Practitioners who recall that era once thought of CPB as dangerous. However, CPB has evolved greatly since those days and has made modern heart surgery possible. With enormous advances in technology over the past twenty years and the development of a branch of medicine called "perfusion," CPB today is very safe, even for infants who weigh fewer than 4 lbs (2 kgs). Most modern heart centers that perform pediatric cardiac surgery have "perfusionists" who are as experienced and skilled at controlling the CPB machine for small babies as are the surgeons at repairing the defects.

CPB is essentially a tool and a "safety net." Babies who are supported during heart surgery by placing them on a heart/lung machine have their circulation maintained while the surgical team dedicates their attention to the operative repair. Any time the surgeon plans on opening the heart to work inside it, CPB probably will be preferred. Although some older techniques for open-heart surgery were often selected in the 1950s and 1960s to avoid relying on CPB, these techniques are more hazardous than modern-day CPB and would only be used today in very unusual cases.

A heart/lung machine takes blood from the body just as it enters the heart, oxygenates the blood, and then returns it to the body on the other side of the heart—thus bypassing the heart and lungs (hence cardiopulmonary bypass). With the heart and lungs "bypassed" and therefore empty of blood, the surgeon can work with a good view of the heart defect and with sufficient time (while the machine supports the circulation) to perform an accurate repair. Furthermore, since the heart no longer needs to work as a pump while the child is on bypass, the heart can actually be stopped (or arrested) during the time of operative repair, therefore further improving the working environment for the surgical team. (Think of how much easier it is to hit a target when it isn't moving.)

There are very few complications related to cardiopulmonary bypass, which is remarkable considering the complexity of the technology. To be placed on CPB, a patient must be given a medicine (heparin) that will prevent blood from clotting when it is exposed to the tubing and other elements of the bypass circuit. During surgery, any bleeding that occurs isn't a problem because the heparinized blood can simply be suctioned into the bypass machine and returned to the patient. Following CPB, after all the tubes used to attach the patient to CPB have been removed, the heparin is "reversed" with another medicine (protamine). Occasionally it is difficult to reverse the heparin effect and patients can have prolonged bleeding following surgery. This may be augmented by the fact that the heart/lung machine can damage platelets (small constituents of blood that aid in clot formation). Postbypass bleeding is most common in tiny babies and in older children who have been cyanotic. In serious cases of ongoing bleeding, blood transfusions are sometimes necessary, and, rarely, the patient will need to go back to the operating room to identify the source of bleeding and correct it.

CPB also seems to induce an "inflammatory" response by the body. This means that some patients (especially small babies) can have generalized swelling of their bodies, and this may take several days following CPB to resolve. This swelling also can affect the lungs, and for this reason some babies will need to remain on a breathing machine for several days following exposure to CPB.

Despite this, CPB is a remarkable tool. Without it, children would still be dying from congenital heart defects. Instead, babies born today with congenital heart disease have a chance at life, and oftentimes that life can be one that is normal from the standpoint of their heart.

What is hypothermia? Is it used in all surgeries? What are the possible complications from it?

Dr. Ungerleider: Normothermia refers to normal body temperature. This is 98.6° Fahrenheit (or 37° Centigrade). Many medical centers will use Centigrade instead of Fahrenheit. *Hyperthermia* refers to temperatures above normal. Temperatures above 38.5°C (101.3°F) are usually considered to be a "fever." *Hypothermia* is a term used to describe temperatures below normal. Obviously there are varying "degrees" of hypothermia. When physicians use the term "mild" hypothermia, they are usually referring to temperatures between 29° and 36°C. "Moderate" hypothermia usually implies temperatures between 23° and 28°C. "Profound" or "deep" hypothermia usually indicates temperatures between 15° and 22°C. These guidelines may vary from institution to institution.

Hypothermia is often used in conjunction with cardiac surgery, with or without the use of cardiopulmonary bypass. There are several reasons why surgeons combine hypothermia with cardiac procedures. As temperature is lowered, metabolism is slowed, and the body needs less oxygen. Since circulation to certain organs may be impaired while the heart and its major vessels are repaired, there is an advantage to using hypothermia. When bypass is not used, mild hypothermia can be achieved by keeping the room cool and allowing the child to "drift" toward 34°-35°C. When a patient is on cardiopulmonary bypass, the blood moving through the machine can be circulated through a heat exchanger and cooled toward whichever "target" temperature the surgical team desires. Most cardiac operations employ some degree of hypothermia to "protect" the body from the "abnormal" circulation of bypass. Relatively short operations (such as closure of atrial or ventricular septal defects) usually employ mild hypothermia. More complicated, longer procedures (such as aortic valve replacement) are usually performed using moderate hypothermia. In longer operations, moderate hypothermia helps to keep the heart from warming, and this improves its ability to tolerate the "stress" of a longer operation. For complex operations in infants, deep hypothermia gives the surgeon the option of slowing blood flow through the pump and still having enough blood circulating through the body to meet oxygen demands. This may be particularly important in certain operations when a normal amount of circulating blood can obscure the surgical field during critical portions of the operation. In some cases it is necessary (or helpful) for the surgeon to stop the circulation entirely. This is referred to as deep hypothermic circulatory arrest. At profoundly hypothermic temperatures, this can be safe for fairly long periods of time—up to an hour, and perhaps longer if certain additional strategies are utilized. Although these are special cases, the use of some degree of hypothermia expands the options available to the surgeon to perform an accurate and safe operative repair of a child's heart defect.

It is difficult to ascribe complications to hypothermia. The process of cooling and then rewarming a patient does take time, and this increases the time that a patient needs to stay on cardiopulmonary bypass. However, the additional time on bypass (especially compared to the advantages of hypothermia) probably does not create any problems. Sometimes patients are removed from bypass while they are still mildly hypothermic. When this is done (to limit bypass time), patients will gradually warm on their own.

"Surgery always seems to take longer than expected. Even if the actual operation is only thirty to forty-five minutes, it may take hours before they get to that point. Inserting IVs, especially in small babies, always seems to take longer than anticipated. Having a nurse come out every hour or so and keeping us posted on the progress of the surgery was helpful to keep us from needlessly worrying that something was going wrong. I think having other family members in the room waiting with us and talking about every-

day things was helpful to pass the time and keep our imaginations from taking over."

—Sara Daniel, mom to Alex (tricuspid atresia, ASD, VSD)

"[During surgery] I would wonder that here she is going through surgery
while other children are being children, which is very difficult to understand
when it's your child in the surgery room."

—Brian Susnis, dad to Taylor (VSD and interrupted aortic arch)

Why can't my child eat before his surgery?

Dr. Ungerleider: The agents used for anesthesia may make a child nau-
seated. If there is food, or any liquid in the stomach, this may be vomited
and could cause choking. If some of the food or liquid is "aspirated" into
the lungs during this choking, this could lead to pneumonia following
surgery. Therefore children may not eat after a prescribed time prior to
elective surgery.

My cardiologist told me there are different ways to fix an ASD (atrial septum defect) now. What are they, and how do I know which one is best for my child?

Dr. Laks: ASDs are the simplest of congenital heart defects and usually
repaired electively during the preschool years. These defects are between
the right and the left atria. The most important reasons for repair are the
benefit of optimal exercise tolerance later in life and to avoid pulmonary
high blood pressure later in life. These defects are also fixed to avoid the
very rare occurrence of a small blood clot traveling from the veins of the
body to the brain instead of the lungs, which are the natural filter of the body
and which dissolve such clots before they cause any damage. The defects
are generally closed by using an incision in the middle of the body going
through the sternum. However, more recently there has been a trend to repair these defects through a much smaller cosmetically appealing incision
through the ribs on the right side of the body. This incision, although more
painful, may allow for a faster return to normal activities during the postoperative period, since it isn't necessary to wait for the bone of the breastplate
to heal. In a more innovative and unproven approach the cardiologist posi-
tions small devices against the defect to close it, thus avoiding surgery alto-
gether. Such devices are currently investigational and being tested under the
guidelines of the Food and Drug Administration. They are not widely available, and the long-term results of such an approach have not been proven.

How do you decide where you make an incision?

Dr. Ungerleider: This decision will be made by your surgeon. Some operations must be performed through the side (between the ribs)—called a "thoracotomy." These usually include repair of coarctation or ligation of a patent ductus arteriosus. Most cardiac operations usually call for a "sternotomy," a vertical incision in the midline and splitting of the breastbone (sternum). Some cardiac operations can be performed through a thoracotomy or a sternotomy (such as closure of an atrial septal defect or placement of a shunt). Reasons for choosing an incision usually relate to what the surgeon feels will enable the procedure to be performed in the best manner. However, in cases where either approach can be used, factors such as which will be most cosmetic, safer, or provide for better options in the future (if future surgery may be required) may influence the decision.

Dr. Laks: In most situations there is no real choice in the incision—cardiac surgery is usually performed through an incision in the middle of the chest. This incision, although not cosmetically appealing, is safe and provides optimal exposure to all the structures of the heart. It implies that the surgeon must cut through the sternum, which is the central bone in front of the chest. Because this incision does not cut muscle and because at the end of the operation the skin is supported by the closure of the bone, which is done with wires, it is one of the least painful incisions in the body. A more cosmetically appealing approach is to make an incision along the ribs. Certain defects are repaired through the ribs on the left side [e.g., aortic coarctation]. There are other defects that can be repaired through the front of the chest or through the ribs on the right side of the body, most commonly defects of the atrial septum and defects of the mitral valve. An incision through the ribs involves cutting muscle and spreading the ribs, which cause more pain during the postoperative period. These incisions have become more popular because of the trend toward a less invasive approach. Approaches through the ribs may allow a quicker recovery and return to normal activities in the first few weeks after surgery, since it isn't necessary to wait for the sternum to heal.

Another approach is the submammary incision, which involves raising the skin at the level of the breast crease across the chest. A skin flap is then elevated, and the bone in front of the chest, the sternum, is then cut in the usual fashion and the heart is accessed normally. This incision may be used to repair very simple defects in which it is predicted that the risk of postoperative complications or the need for repeat surgery in the future is minimal. This incision is cosmetically appealing since it will be completely invisible unless the entire chest is exposed. It is preferable for girls because the incision will be hidden. The incision will be visible for boys and generally is not recommended.

What difference, if any, does it make in terms of recovery postoperatively?

Dr. Ungerleider: Older patients who can communicate and who have had both a thoracotomy and a sternotomy often claim that a thoracotomy is more painful for the initial few days following surgery. A thoracotomy may lead to numbness in the side and can even lead to numbness in the breast. It also can lead to scarring (and deformity) of the breast tissue as it develops in a young woman unless the incision is made low enough. Long-term patients who have had thoracotomies can develop curvature (scoliosis) of the spine. A sternotomy has very few complications. It is a more noticeable incision and therefore more difficult for the patient to "hide." A sternotomy can be performed with a horizontal skin incision that is made low, below the breasts, and in some cases where cosmetics are important, this is an option. The best approach is to discuss options with the surgeon, but to be amenable to whatever incision he or she recommends, since the surgeon usually will recommend the incision he or she feels is safest for your child while enabling the surgeon to perform the best operation.

"This occurred in 1991, when Beth was five years old and in the hospital for her second open-heart surgery. She watched a lot of TV (in the hospital). She had a pacemaker inserted eleven days after her open-heart surgery, and the first thing she said when she awoke after the pacemaker surgery was 'Where's the remote control?' "

—Kathy Grampovnik, mom to Beth (aortic stenosis, subvalvular aortic stenosis, surgical heart block with a pacemaker)

"Jason had a camera follow him through his most recent surgery, beginning with the preop room and continuing until he was discharged from the hospital! (He plans on using it for a future biology project!)"

—WenDee Riley, mom to Jason (transposition of the great vessels)

Heart Valves

My daughter has a problem with one of her valves. How do you decide when to fix a valve and when to replace it?

Dr. Laks: In general, it's preferable to fix a valve rather than to replace it. This is more important when it's anticipated that the child will grow and that any artificial valve placed will have to be replaced with a larger-size valve. The other issue of major importance is that artificial valves require the child to take blood thinners permanently. Although valves that come from animals require only aspirin as a blood thinner, mechanical valves, which are most commonly made of pyrolytic carbon [synthetic black diamonds], require anticoagulation with Coumadin. Although mechanical valves have the advantage of being bench-tested for the past hundred years, blood-thinning regimens can lead to bleeding complications such as easy bruising during contact sports. Further, women who want to get pregnant should avoid Coumadin. To avoid these problems, surgeons have used homografts to replace valves in children. Homografts are valves that come from other humans and have been frozen to be preserved. They last slightly longer than valves that come from animals but are not always available in all sizes. A valve repair is preferable even if it means a second valve repair or a valve replacement in ten or fifteen years. The additional repair delays the need for a valve replacement and potential complications associated with a valve replacement.

Dr. Ungerleider: In general, it's preferable to repair rather than replace a valve. It's also important that whatever a surgeon does to a valve, its function be significantly improved by the operative procedure. It's not desirable to repair a valve and have it require surgery again within months or even a couple of years. This is not always avoidable, and if your surgeon thinks that he or she can provide an adequate valve repair, he or she probably will choose that option and hope, along with you, that the repair will withstand the forces of the heart's powerful contractions and function well for a long time.

If a surgeon doesn't feel confident that he or she can produce an adequate valve repair, then he or she may select to replace the valve. Several factors enter into this decision. If your child is small and still growing, it may be preferable to provide the best repair possible until your child is bigger and able to accept a replacement valve that he or she will be less likely to outgrow. Some heart valves are more "important" than others, and therefore it is more critical that they function well. This would encourage a decision favoring replacement rather than "tolerable" repair of those valves. The valves on the left side of the heart—the aortic and mitral valves—are more important in this way. Patients can live quite well without a pulmonary valve or with a leaking tricuspid valve on the right side of the heart. Finally, the outcome for artificial valves in various locations of the heart vary, as do the options for valve replacements, and this affects surgical decision-making.

The mitral valve is the valve that lends itself best to repair, and there are several techniques that a surgeon can employ to improve mitral valve function. Furthermore, there are very few options for mitral valve replacement. In most cases the only alternative is a mechanical valve that will require a lifetime of blood thinners and some restrictions on activity. Therefore the surgeon might try very hard to repair a mitral valve if at all possible.

The aortic valve doesn't lend itself very well to repair other than dilatations to enlarge its opening. Although an occasional leaking aortic valve can be repaired, the outcome for these types of procedures has not been very satisfying, and most surgeons would elect to replace an aortic valve that is severely defective. Furthermore, there are several good options for aortic valve replacement, including the pulmonary autograft (Ross) procedure, or the use of aortic homografts in addition to the various prosthetic valves available.

What are the different types of replacement valves? What are the advantages and disadvantages of each? How do you decide which is right for my child?

Dr. Ungerleider: Heart valves are mechanical (metal) or tissue. There are a number of companies that manufacture mechanical heart valves, but the ones in most common use in this country are the "bileaflet" design (St. Jude or Carbomedics). These valves have leaflets that are hinged onto an outer "annular" ring so they open in only one direction. The annular ring, in turn, is covered with soft felt material through which sutures can be passed. Because these valves are made of extremely sophisticated materials, they have very reliable function and durability. They are relatively easy for surgeons to implant and for this reason are a popular choice by many groups who offer heart valve replacement surgery. These metal valves could conceivably last for decades, but because they present an artificial surface to the blood, it is possible that small clots can form around the hinge mechanisms or the "sewing ring." Therefore children who have metal valves need to take blood thinners (anticoagulants) for the remainder of their life as long as they still have the mechanical valve in place. This may impose significant limitations on lifestyle, since patients on anticoagulation must refrain from various forms of activity (such as skiing, horseback riding, contact sports, or anything where a fall or a sharp blow to the head or body is possible). Along with anticoagulation comes a lifelong risk of complications related to the anticoagulation, including stroke or a serious bleeding event. This risk has been estimated at between 1 and 2 percent per patient year, meaning that over thirty years a patient has a 30 to 60 percent likelihood of a serious neurologic or bleeding complication. Furthermore, mechanical valves have a persistent risk of infection or of developing a "leak" around the sewing ring that might necessitate reoperation. Mechanical valves do not grow and in small sizes can produce some obstruction to blood flow, especially during exercise. For these reasons, decisions for placement of mechanical valves must be individualized to specific patients and anatomic location.

Mechanical valves are best suited for placement in the mitral position, since currently there are no better options for pediatric patients. It is arguable whether a mechanical valve is a preferred option for the aortic or the tricuspid position; those issues would need to be discussed with your child's care providers.

Tissue valves come in several forms. For years the most common tissue (biologic) valves were those manufactured from the valve tissue of pigs or from the pericardium (sac that lines the heart) of cows. This tissue was "fixed" with gluteraldehyde and encircled by a "sewing ring." These valves were also easy for surgeons to implant, and because they aren't mechanical, they don't require anticoagulation. When first introduced, it appeared that they would provide children with a wonderful alternative to mechanical valves. Unfortunately, it has been discovered that biologic tissue valves can degenerate very rapidly in children and in some cases may need to be replaced within a couple of years. Despite their initial attractiveness, they are now rarely used for pediatric valve replacement except for valves on the right side of the heart (tricuspid and pulmonary), where they have several advantages and are preferred by several groups.

Over the past fifteen to twenty years, another type of tissue valve has become popular—human tissue valves, which are called homografts (or allografts). Donated by people after they die, homografts are now frozen and kept in freezers in the operating rooms of surgeons who use these valves. Both aortic and pulmonary homografts are available. Clearly, human valves have the best possible design, but their implantation takes more training and experience than for mechanical or biologic valves. Consequently not all surgeons use them. Homografts can be placed in the pulmonary or aortic position. They don't require anticoagulation. Patients with homograft valves in the aortic or pulmonary position rarely have restrictions placed on their lifestyles and can exercise vigorously. Although the body does not "reject" homograft valve tissue, homografts are not living tissue and will degenerate over time. Therefore it is predicted that homografts in the aortic position may last fifteen to twenty years. Due to the lower pressures of the pulmonary circulation, pulmonary homografts theoretically could last longer. Because homografts are not living tissue, they will not grow and, when placed in a small child, may need to be replaced as the child outgrows this valve. It is also possible to "transplant" a patient's own pulmonary valve to his or her aortic position (pulmonary autograft), and this does provide them with a living, growing, normal valve in the aortic position. The pulmonary valve area is reconstructed with a human pulmonary homograft (Ross Procedure). This option is discussed later in this chapter (see "Types of Surgical Procedures").

Deciding which of these valves to use is complex and relates to several factors, including the age and size of the child, the anatomic position that requires valve replacement, the lifestyle of the child, and the preference of the surgical team. In general, the tricusipid valve can be replaced with either a mechanical or a biologic valve, but not with a homograft. The pulmonary valve can be replaced with a homograft or a biologic valve. Mitral valve replacement in children usually requires a mechanical valve (there is some investigation with the use of homografts in this area). Aortic valve replacement can be performed with the pulmonary autograft, an aortic homograft, or with a mechanical valve. Biologic valves are not recommended for aortic valve replacement in children.

Do you expect there to be significant advances in the types of valves available over the next decade?

Dr. Ungerleider: Advances with tissue engineering may make it possible to "grow" heart valves for individual patients using their own tissue. This will provide essentially normal, living valves for individual patients. However, this technology is not available now.

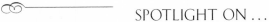

SPOTLIGHT ON ...
Rashida and Raghu Mendu, founders,
The Heart of a Child Foundation

When Rashida and Raghu Mendu lost their daughter Samara to complex congenital heart disease in 1996, they immediately felt they needed to do something to honor her. They reluctantly agreed to a memorial service and were surprised when 120 people attended. Many of these people wanted to send flowers, but the Mendus thought it would be more useful if they made a donation in Samara's name to UCLA Medical Center, where Samara had all of her treatment. Their friends came through with more than $20,000.

The Mendus then started looking for a way to contribute money toward something in the field of pediatric cardiology. They started talking with some doctors. And what they found was that because research funding was so hard to get and researchers, particularly in pediatrics, tended to be so poorly compensated, science was losing some of its brightest minds. That's when Rashida and Raghu decided to start a foundation that would honor Samara's memory as well as provide research funds to further the doctors' knowledge of pediatric cardiology.

First called the Samara Foundation, they changed the name to the Heart of a Child Foundation to broaden the appeal and to make it clearer what the foundation was all about. They were bolstered early in 1998 when Sylvester Stallone, whose daughter, Sophia, also had heart surgery at UCLA, donated $200,000 to the foundation and again later that year when they were named one of the two official charities for the World Polo Championships in Santa Barbara. The World Polo Championships were accompanied by a fund-raiser for the Heart of a Child Foundation at the House of Blues in Los Angeles.

Rashida and Raghu are busy promoting the foundation. Neither draws a salary, with Raghu working for the foundation full-time (Rashida cut back her hours after the February 1998 birth of daughter Jihana Samaya). Their hope is to build the foundation into a national organization with chapters in several cities. They would like to raise enough money to begin to endow professorships in pediatric cardiology. And the foundation recently formed a small suborganization called Little Hearts on the Mend, dedicated to helping children in other countries come to the United States to get medical treatment.

If you would like to make a donation or would like additional information about the foundation, please feel free to write to Rashida and Raghu at:

> The Heart of a Child Foundation
> 26710 Fond du Lac Road
> Rancho Palos Verdes, CA 90275

Types of Surgical Procedures

What is the difference between open and closed heart surgery?

Dr. Laks: Open-heart surgery implies that during the operation the child will be placed on the heart/lung machine. This machine is used in every open-heart operation in the world and diverts the blood from the heart and the lungs and puts it back into the body after fulfilling the function of the heart and the lungs. This allows the surgeon to operate in a bloodless field "inside the heart." The term "open" refers to the fact that, following the operation, air that was introduced during opening of the heart must be evacuated prior to weaning off the heart/lung machine. The heart/lung machine is an unnatural route for blood to pass through and therefore has certain side effects that may take several days to subside in the postoperative period. This is why a child may require use of a mechanical ventilator for a short period of time after surgery.

A "closed" heart procedure is generally one in which the heart/lung machine is not used; this limits the extent of surgery. Side effects of the heart/lung machine don't occur in such situations, but the alternative is that the repair may not be as complete. The heart/lung machine has been used routinely since the late 1950s.

What is the difference between partial and definitive repair?

Dr. Laks: A definitive repair implies that normal anatomy and function have been restored. In the previous era there were many instances when surgery would restore normal function but not normal anatomy. This was a good solution to many problems. However, such situations would lead to complications fifteen or twenty years after the operation. Today surgeons strive to restore normal anatomy and normal function as much as possible. Children may require further surgery such as valve changes as they grow, but the repair of their original defect is permanent. There are other occasions when partial repair may be indicated to have a more staged approach toward a definitive repair. For example, a child may be so small and the required surgery so complex that it's better to do it in stages. If there are several defects, although it may be possible to repair them all at once, it may be safer to repair them in stages with several procedures. There are yet other situations where, for example, one may wait for the pulmonary arteries to grow to reconstruct them more completely. In such a situation, the surgeon will consider a partial repair to enhance this growth.

Why are some surgeries done in stages? Why can't you fix everything at once?

Dr. Ungerleider: Decisions regarding whether to provide complete, single-stage repair versus staged repair depend on the type of procedure, the condition of the patient at the time of surgery, and the anatomy of the heart defect. In some cases decisions are made in accordance with the "comfort" of the surgical team with the type of surgery required.

Patients with single ventricles who will require Fontan procedures must be repaired in stages. The flow dynamics (physiology) of the Fontan procedure require progressive stages designed to allow the pulmonary arteries to grow, protect the pulmonary arteries from high pressure, and allow the child's physiology to adapt gradually.

Patients with otherwise repairable heart defects can undergo complete repair in infancy or palliation in infancy, with repair at a later time depending on the specifics of the situation. In some cases palliative operations are performed with complete repair reserved for a later time. This will be true if portions of the anatomy have to be prepared for repair (such as "growing" pulmonary arteries) or if repair might require placement of material (such as a homograft) for which it might be desirable to have the patient attain a larger size. Sometimes infants with repairable defects have other problems that increase their risk of complete repair, and palliation is performed. Some surgical teams prefer patients to attain a certain size or age before they feel comfortable offering complete repair; these patients will receive palliation if something needs to be done before they reach that target age or weight.

My child has hypoplastic left heart syndrome. Why do some doctors recommend transplant and others recommend three staged repairs? What are the advantages and disadvantages of each?

Dr. Ungerleider: Children with hypoplastic left heart syndrome (HLHS) are born without the pumping chamber to the body and consequently must be staged to a Fontan procedure. Furthermore, this Fontan procedure needs to be "based" on the right ventricle as the systemic pump. Results with the first stage (Norwood procedure) for HLHS were poor in most centers. Historically, children with Fontan procedures that were based on the right ventricle had poor outcomes (with respect to quality of life) even if they survived.

Cardiac transplantation seemed to be an appropriate alternative to these "bad" Fontans. A successful transplant provides the child with a "normal" heart and a quality of life that might be preferable.

Unfortunately, as more surgeons became interested in infant heart transplantation, donor hearts became even scarcer and babies would wait several weeks or months for an organ. Many of these babies died waiting. Those who did get transplants faced a life filled with the "complications" of heart transplantation—multiple hospital visits to control episodes of rejection, an increased risk of developing certain types of cancer or serious infections, and the late (seven to ten years after transplant) occurrence of coronary artery disease necessitating repeat transplantation.

Concurrently, several surgical groups became more successful with the staging procedures, and techniques improved so that patients survive with relatively normal functional outcomes. Because of the balance between organ unavailability and improved outcomes with the Norwood procedure, randomized clinical trials indicate similar survival rates for these treatment modalities. Most often, patients will be offered both options, but centers that are successful with the staging procedures will usually prefer them, since staging to Fontan doesn't require the patient to wait for weeks in an intensive care unit. Furthermore, heart transplantation is always an option for these patients years down the road if they begin to have problems related to their Fontan. Perhaps by that time some of the problems currently associated with transplantation will be solved.

"The most difficult thing that I have faced is seeing my child almost die at one week old. My husband and I decided that we would go with three staged surgeries rather than a heart transplant for our son. The first night, as we watched our child nearly die, I wondered if we had done the right thing."

—*Deanna Smith, mom to Nicholas (HLHS)*

What is pulmonary artery banding? When is it used?

Dr. Laks: Pulmonary artery banding refers to a process where the circulation in the lungs is purposely limited. This procedure can be used in several situations. Formerly, when a child had a heart defect that permitted too much blood to pass through the lungs, the child would frequently develop respiratory infections and have difficulty breathing during strenuous activities. Additionally, excess circulation in the lungs will lead to permanent high blood pressure after a period of time. The lungs actually have a much lower blood pressure than the body, particularly after the first three months of life. Such a situation would then preclude a more definitive repair. A banding procedure may be used to stage a complex definitive repair and to protect the lungs from excess blood flow. In such a situation, a child may leave surgery with "oxygen saturation" in the 75–85 percent range. The normal oxygen saturation is 100 percent, but since the lungs are being protected from excess blood flow during the operation, the post-operative oxygen saturation would be less than 100 percent. In this case when there is excess blood flow the oxygen saturation never goes higher than 100 percent but the lungs are not being protected.

Pulmonary artery banding is performed less frequently now that surgeons have become more comfortable with a more definitive surgery during the first year of life. It remains a useful tool in certain situations that require a staged approach. The most important example of this situation is a child who will ultimately not have a left side and a right side of the heart but only a single ventricle. When these children are in the first months of life, the single ventricle is used to pump blood into both the lungs and the rest of the body. To balance this blood flow and to protect the lungs against overcirculation [since this is the pathway of least resistance], a band may be placed around the pulmonary artery to increase the resistance mechanically and to protect the lungs from overcirculation. As the child gets older and the lungs mature, the child can then proceed to a reconstruction in which the veins of the body are connected directly to the arteries to the lungs. This eliminates a need for the right side of the heart. This is known as the Fontan procedure. It is impossible to perform the Fontan procedure if the lungs have not been protected from overcirculation and develop a high resistance. The pulmonary artery band is extremely important in children who are eventually destined to have the Fontan procedure.

What is an arterial switch? When is it used?

Dr. Laks: An arterial switch operation is an operation used for a condition called transposition of the great arteries. This is a situation where the right side of the heart pumps the blood into the body, and the left side of the heart pumps the blood into the lungs. This is an abnormal situation and is reversed from the normal situation in which the circulation of the lungs and the rest of the body are in "series" rather than in "parallel." Children with such a diagnosis cannot survive unless there is mixing of the blood inside the heart caused by another defect (atrial or ventricle septal defect).

Previously, a physiological correction called the atrial switch operation was performed. During this operation, the entrance to the right and left ventricles (the atria) would be reversed so that the right ventricle would pump the blood into the body after receiving its inflow from the left atrium. The left ventricle would pump blood into the lungs after receiving its inflow from the right atrium. The right atrium receives the blue unoxygenated blood from the body. This was a good repair; however, the right ventricle wasn't optimal when it came to its ability to pump blood into the body over a lifetime. Nature has designed the right ventricle to pump the blood into a much lower-resistance system—the pulmonary circulation.

Since the 1970s, as surgeons have gained more experience in cardiac surgery and coronary artery manipulations, it has become possible to perform the arterial switch procedure. During this operation, the two vessels that exit the heart toward the lungs and the rest of the body respectively are literally cut, switched, and then sewed back on. This involves manipulation of the coronary arteries—an extremely delicate procedure. It is usually performed in the first three weeks of life when the left ventricle is trained to pump blood against the high resistance seen in the pulmonary circulation. The resistance in the pulmonary circulation falls after several weeks of life, and the arterial switch can no longer be performed in one stage after this time. A pulmonary artery band must then be added to mechanically increase the resistance against which the left ventricle is pumping so that the muscle of the heart may be "trained" to pump against the high resistance in the body. Normally the systemic circulation always has a higher resistance than the pulmonary circulation, except in the first four weeks of life, when the resistance is equal. It then falls until the end of the third month of life, as the lungs mature.

What is an intra-atrial baffle procedure? When is it used? Is it the same as a Mustard or Senning procedure?

Dr. Laks: An intra-atrial baffle is used to divert blood from the left atrium to the right ventricle and from the right atrium to the left ventricle. In the previous era, this was a common procedure to restore normal physiology, but it did not address the issue of restoring normal anatomy. The right ventricle is shaped and structured to pump blood against the low resistance of pulmonary circulation. Because it has a high reserve, it can be used to pump blood in the systemic circulation—a much higher resistance. One can anticipate that this could work for several years, but there is a risk that after ten or twenty years the ventricle may fail, particularly as a child grows and makes more demands on it. Alternatively, the ventricle may have sufficient strength to pump the blood during a child's resting state but not during exercise. As a result, the child may have to limit some activities. Ultimately, if such physiology should fail, a child would need a heart transplant operation. Currently every effort is being made to avoid such a baffle procedure (also known as Mustard or Senning procedures). The arterial switch procedure is more commonly used to ensure that the left ventricle, which is designed to pump blood against a high resistance, is in fact a systemic ventricle as nature would normally have it.

There are very rare instances when such operations are still carried out. These are exceptional.

What is a Ross procedure?

Dr. Ungerleider: The Ross procedure is named for Mr. Donald Ross, a cardiac surgeon from London who has been a pioneer for the use of human valves for aortic valve replacement. (In England, surgeons are referred to as "Mr." rather than "Dr.") Mr. Ross believes that the best valve for replacement of a defective valve is a human valve—donated by a person at death. These valves, called homografts, can be frozen, and then thawed in the operating room when they are needed. A homograft isn't "living" tissue, but it can function well for many years before it degenerates. Because it's a normal aortic valve, when implanted in the aortic position it can allow the patient to lead an essentially normal life, with very few if any limitations. Although a homograft isn't "rejected" like living organs, it will not grow. Furthermore, usually it will last only fifteen to twenty years. For these last two reasons, it may not be optimal for very young, growing patients.

In 1967 Mr. Ross was confronted with a patient who needed an aortic valve replacement. He excised the defective aortic valve and prepared a homograft for implantation in the aortic position, only to have it accidentally destroyed by some of the operating room equipment. He had been thinking about doing an operation that suddenly became necessary—the operation that now carries his name. All of us have a valve on the right side of our heart that is structurally just like an aortic valve. This valve leads from the heart to the lungs and is called the pulmonary valve. Although it's impossible to live without a functioning aortic valve, it's possible to live without a pulmonary valve. This is because the blood pressure in the lungs is much less than in the rest of the body. Mr. Ross removed this patient's pulmonary valve and placed it in the more important aortic position. This pulmonary valve was the patient's own, normal, living valve and is called an autograft. Although he didn't do so in his first patient, he began replacing the pulmonary valve with a homograft.

The "pulmonary autograft" operation to replace a defective aortic valve is the Ross procedure. It is now performed throughout this country by pediatric heart surgeons with excellent results. It has the advantage of providing a child with a normal, growing aortic valve that should allow him or her to have a normal lifestyle. The homograft in the pulmonary position, which replaces the pulmonary valve that was removed for the aorta, can last a very long time on this low-pressure side of the heart, and may not even be critical for survival. The Ross procedure is now becoming the procedure of choice at many children's heart centers for aortic valve replacement in children (and even for adults up to sixty years old!).

What is a Blalock-Taussig shunt? When is it used?

Dr. Ungerleider: Alfred Blalock was the chief of surgery at Johns Hopkins Medical Center in the 1940s. He is considered to be one of the pioneers of modern heart surgery. Helen Taussig was the chief of pediatric cardiology at Hopkins during the same era. She also is considered to be one of the pioneers of how we treat congenital heart disease today. In 1940, cardiopulmonary bypass wasn't available, and many children with serious congenital heart defects died. For those children who survived, very little could be done. This was especially frustrating in the case of older children who survived infancy with their heart defect, only to be hospitalized when they were several years old with severe manifestations of congenital heart disease. One of the most compelling signs of congenital heart disease was apparent in those children who had very little blood going to their lungs. Since they couldn't oxygenate their blood, they had a very dusky appearance and were called "blue babies."

In his laboratory, Dr. Blalock had been experimenting with ways to get blood from the rest of the body into the lungs. He did this by cutting the artery to the arm (the subclavian artery, without which the arm would still survive) and connecting it to the arteries leading to the lungs. On one fateful day in 1944, a small child with the heart defect called tetralogy of Fallot presented to the cardiology service at Johns Hopkins. In this heart defect there is a large hole in the heart and a very narrow opening between the heart and the lungs. Instead of going to the lungs to get oxygenated, blood has an "easier" time going through the hole in the wall that separates the two sides of the heart and being pumped directly to the body—without oxygen. These babies can be quite "blue." Helen Taussig approached Dr. Blalock and asked if his experiments had progressed to where he would be willing to try his subclavian artery "shunt" procedure on a child, because without some treatment, the child she was seeing that day would surely die. In a landmark operation, Dr. Blalock performed the first "extracardiac, palliative" procedure for a congenital heart defect. He did precisely what he had been working on in his laboratory—he divided the child's subclavian artery and connected it to the pulmonary artery (artery to the lung). This enabled some blood that had been pumped to the body to travel to the lungs to get oxygen. The child survived and was much improved. With this operation the field of pediatric cardiac surgery was "born." Surgeons now had a therapy, albeit temporary, but nevertheless something helpful that they could offer to these extremely sick and dying children. This direct connection ("shunt") between the subclavian artery and the pulmonary artery has ever since been termed the Blalock-Taussig shunt.

Today the term "shunt" is applied to any connection between the systemic (aortic) circulation and the pulmonary (lung) circulation. Over the years, a large variety of shunts have been developed by several surgeons. In almost all cases, shunts are used for infants with inadequate pulmonary blood flow as a way to increase blood flow to the lungs and thus oxygenation of the blood. Since shunts don't correct the cardiac defect but rather provide a more stable situation for some later, more definitive procedure, the use of shunts is termed palliation. The Blalock-Taussig shunt is rarely used today. Instead of dividing the subclavian artery, surgeons often use a graft of artificial material and interpose it between the subclavian and pulmonary arteries. This preserves the subclavian artery and serves the purposes intended for the shunt very nicely. This type of shunt, which can be inserted through a thoracotomy (incision in the side) or through a sternotomy (incision in the midline), is called a modified Blalock-Taussig (or BT) shunt.

Shunts create a situation whereby the heart actually works harder. The chamber pumping blood to the body now also pumps the shunt circulation and can be working two to three times the normal amount (depending upon the size and amount of blood going through the shunt). The heart actually tolerates this quite well, especially since the shunt provides improved oxygenation. Since a shunt is palliative, it is usually the intention of the surgeon to have the shunt serve a purpose (e.g., help the pulmonary arteries to grow or to create stable flow to the lungs) until a more definitive procedure can be performed, usually several months and often within a year following placement of the shunt.

What is a Glenn shunt? When is it used?

Dr. Ungerleider: Considering the discussion above regarding the term "shunt," it is probably a misnomer to call a Glenn procedure a "shunt." However, various care providers often call it a Glenn shunt; therefore you should be familiar with the procedure that is referred to in this way.

The Glenn procedure is a connection between the superior vena cava (SVC) and the pulmonary arteries. The original procedure as described by Dr. William Glenn was a connection between the SVC and the right pulmonary artery. Today almost all Glenn procedures are connections between the SVC and both pulmonary arteries ("bidirectional Glenn"). The Glenn procedure, as it is used today, is sometimes called a "cavopulmonary anastomosis," and this is much more descriptive. (You may also hear the term "HemiFontan" from your cardiology and surgery team. Essentially, a "HemiFontan" is a method of performing a bidirectional Glenn procedure.)

This procedure is used as a way to improve blood flow to the lungs, but it has a critical difference compared to other "shunt" procedures. The SVC carries unoxygenated blood returning to the heart from the upper body. (Blood from the lower body returns to the heart via the inferior vena cava or IVC. The SVC and the IVC are the two veins that bring all the blood back to the heart from the rest of the body.) In the Glenn anastomosis, the blood in the SVC is diverted into the pulmonary circulation without having to travel through the heart. In this sense, a Glenn anastomosis provides a form of "right heart bypass." Since the blood is not being "pumped" into the pulmonary circulation, this will work only if resistance to blood flow in the lungs is very low. This requires large pulmonary arteries and usually that a child be older than three months.

The advantage of the Glenn is that it removes a lot of work from the heart that has been surviving with a shunt or with a pulmonary artery band. With either of the latter two arrangements, the heart muscle must "pump" extra blood—some of which goes to the lungs (through the shunt or across the PA band) and some of which goes to the rest of the body (through the aorta). Eventually all this extra work can tire the heart muscle. With the Glenn, the heart just pumps blood to the aorta. As this blood returns from the body, the blood coming from the upper body goes through the lungs en route to the heart. The heart, with a Glenn procedure, is receiving oxygenated blood, but does not have to perform extra work to make this happen. For this reason, your care providers might recommend a Glenn procedure after three months of age with "takedown" of any previously constructed shunt or PA band.

The Glenn procedure (cavopulmonary anastomosis) is essentially a "partial Fontan" procedure. The Fontan procedure is discussed in the next section. The Glenn procedure is used as a method of staging a child toward a Fontan procedure. In a sense the Glenn procedure enables the child to "practice" Fontan physiology. It produces a Fontan arrangement for the upper body while allowing the blood from the lower body to continue to travel through the heart.

After a Glenn procedure, your child still will not have normal oxygen levels in his or her blood. Although the blood from the upper body, which traverses the lungs to get back to the heart, will have oxygen, the blood from the lower body does not go through the lungs. When these two pools of blood meet in the heart, the resulting mixture is blood that is partially oxygenated. The typical oxygen saturations following a Glenn procedure are in the range of 78 to 83 percent.

What is the Fontan procedure? When is it used?

Dr. Ungerleider: The Fontan procedure is named for a French surgeon, Francis Fontan, who was among the first to demonstrate how patients who lacked a right ventricle (the chamber that normally pumps blood to the lungs) could still survive by having the veins that return to the heart [superior vena cava (SVC) and inferior vena cava (IVC)] deliver blood directly to the lungs. He determined that for this to work, there were several requirements, which he termed the "Ten Commandments" for a Fontan. These related to pulmonary artery anatomy and resistance, as well as to the efficiency of the heart to fill with blood and pump it forward without high "back pressure." In a sense, the Fontan is like a gravity-fed system of blood flow through the lungs. Without a pump to push blood through the lungs, the blood will flow through the lungs only if there is sort of a "downslope." Increases in pulmonary resistance, or in resistance of the heart (downstream) to accept blood will create a need for higher pressure to "drive" blood through the lungs. Unfortunately the venous system cannot generate very high pressures, and if pulmonary resistance is too high, a Fontan will not work.

The Fontan is a very useful procedure today for patients who are born without a ventricle (either right or left ventricle). It is commonly used for children born with small or absent right ventricles (e.g., tricuspid atresia, pulmonary atresia with intact ventricular septum, Ebstein's anomaly) as well as for children born with small or absent left ventricles (e.g., hypoplastic left heart syndrome, critical aortic stenosis) or those whose ventricles cannot be separated into two (e.g., unbalanced AV canal defects). When the left ventricle is small or absent, then the right ventricle is reconstructed with surgery to become the major pumping chamber to the body. Although not initially intended to perform this function, the right ventricle can be an adequate systemic pump, and children who have Fontan procedures based on a right ventricle (e.g., hypoplastic left heart syndrome) can have a fairly good functional outcome.

The decision to perform a Fontan procedure is generally made soon after a child is born and prior to *any* surgical intervention. Commonly, patients are "staged" to a Fontan. Oftentimes this includes a shunt or a pulmonary artery band in the first days following birth. If the right ventricle needs to be reconstructed as the systemic ventricle, this will be done as part of the initial shunt procedure. Usually children are converted to a bidirectional Glenn at three months to a year old, depending on several factors. The Fontan is generally "complete" between two and three years of age, when the pulmonary arteries have grown well and their resistance to blood flow should be quite low.

In some instances you will hear the term "fenestrated Fontan." Immediately following a Fontan procedure, the blood on the venous side of the circulation will have a fairly high pressure. This is necessary to "push" blood through the pulmonary vascular bed. After a child has received a Fontan completion, the *only* way blood can get back to the heart to be pumped to the body is through the lungs. Unfortunately, cardiopulmonary bypass can transiently increase pulmonary resistance, and it may be hard for the child to generate venous pressures high enough to push blood through the lungs. A small "fenestration" (hole) in the Fontan connection can allow some venous blood to cross over to the pumping side *without* having to flow through the lungs. Although this blood will not have oxygen and this will result in lower oxygen levels for the child, it will augment the blood that is able to travel through the lungs and provide an adequate amount of blood for the pumping chamber to be able to deliver sufficient blood to the body. As pulmonary resistance falls in the days following surgery, blood is more likely to be able to flow through the lungs, and the fenestration becomes less important. These fenestrations often will close off on their own. If not, they may not present any long-term problems, or they can be closed by cardiologists in the catheterization laboratory if necessary. The other advantage of fenestrations is that they reduce the venous pressure necessary for a Fontan to work. When venous pressure gets too high, fluid can leak out of the blood vessels into the space around the lungs (pleural effusions) or into the abdominal cavity (ascites), and this can prolong convalescence following a Fontan.

What types of patches are used to repair holes?

Dr. Ungerleider: Cardiovascular patches all share certain qualities. They are soft so that they won't tear off the muscle of the heart. They are impervious to blood—they don't leak. They must be tough enough to hold suture without tearing or fraying. A variety of materials meet these requirements and are used by various surgeons. It probably doesn't matter what material is used or how it is sewn in place.

When a child's chest is opened for the first time, the heart is contained within a sac of very tough tissue called the pericardium. The pericardium must be opened to enable access to the heart. The heart doesn't need to be enveloped in pericardium, and a portion of this pericardium can be removed and used by the surgeon as patch material. Alternatively, the surgeon can choose from a variety of artificial (prosthetic) materials, including Gore-Tex, Dacron, or Teflon felt.

What happens to the patch as my child grows?

Dr. Ungerleider: After a patch is placed in (or on) the heart, it slowly becomes incorporated into the substance of the heart. The heart will gradually cover the patch with a lining of its own cells (called endothelium). As the patch endothelializes, it becomes less recognizable as a patch. In fact, if you were to look in the heart a year after surgery, you would not be able to easily tell that it contained a patch.

The patch material does not grow, but the rest of the heart does. The patch does its job by closing the hole. Over time, the rest of the heart grows, and eventually, as your child becomes an adult, his or her heart will contain what might be by then a very small and totally endothelialized patch.

What do you recommend to help nervous parents when their child is going into surgery?

Mr. Sklenar: A child's needing surgery can cause anxiety for a parent regardless of the diagnosis or procedure that will be done. There is nothing anyone can say to make you less nervous, and this is a natural response. However, three main points to remember are: Get information, get support, and take care of yourself. Obtaining as much information as you can about the cardiac problem and the procedure that will be done can help decrease some of the anxiety. Make sure you meet with your child's physician and be prepared to ask as many questions as you need. It's a good idea to go to the meeting with a list of prepared questions you have developed with other family members (they may think of something you overlooked). Write the answers to the questions so you can refer to them. It's a good idea to meet with the physician accompanied by a family member or a friend; an extra set of ears can catch what you miss. Take care of yourself so you can take care of your child. Try to rest prior to the surgery, and eat something on the morning of the surgery (even if you're not hungry) to keep your blood sugar level up. Have someone with you at the hospital on the day of the surgery, and be prepared to be patient, since the team will be so focused on taking care of your child that they probably won't be able to give you frequent progress reports until the surgery is over.

What natural methods do you suggest to help parents ease nervousness and remain strong during this kind of ordeal?

Mr. Sklenar: Everyone has his or her own methods of easing stress. Some parents sleep, some pray for inner strength, while others may prefer to eat frequently. Whatever method works for you should have the goal of providing what you need to help yourself, your child, and your family remain strong. Drinking too much coffee or any other beverage with caffeine tends to make one more nervous and "jumpy." Avoid alcohol, which can impair judgment. Remember that your child is in the hospital and is surrounded by qualified healthcare professionals. You need to take care of yourself despite the fact that you may feel guilty about your child going through this experience. Take breaks and allow other family members or friends to visit with your child while you take a refreshing shower, take a walk, run errands, or spend time with your other children (which is very important during this time). Remain informed and ask all of your questions. It's better to ask than to keep the anxiety inside. Sometimes speaking to other families who have gone through this experience can be extremely helpful. If you are interested in this, you should speak with the social worker or the physician, who can facilitate this or inform you about any community or hospital support groups that may be available.

I have heard about children developing heart block as a result of their corrective surgery. What is this, and why does it happen? How often does this complication occur? Why do these children need a pacemaker? Do all children with this condition need a pacemaker?

Dr. Laks: Heart block is common after all forms of open-heart surgery. This is temporary in most cases and is treated with temporary pacemaker wires, which are placed at the time of surgery and are removed when the child goes home. Occasionally, because certain defects occur very close to the nerve tissues of the heart, stitches used to repair the defect can create blockages in these nerves; hence the term heart block. About 2 to 5 percent of children will need a permanent pacemaker due to heart block. The heart has a backup internal rate, which is slower but adequate in case of an emergency. Pacemakers were, in fact, invented in the 1950s and 1960s for children who had repair of heart defects and are considered reliable. They require periodic battery changes, and as technology improves the electrical leads are changed less frequently. Pacemakers are programmable and can increase their rate during exercise by sensing motion and temperature, reproducing the heart's normal response. They never stop. The battery power will slow down progressively over the course of a year. That is why all patients with pacemakers are periodically followed by their cardiologists.

"The hardest thing was knowing that the corrections (repairing the VSDs and ASDs) caused a need for a pacemaker. That was a very hard thing to deal with and accept."

—Shelly Corush, mom to Seth (coarctation of the aortic artery, enlarged pulmonary artery, several ASDs and VSDs, heart block with a pacemaker—as a result of the ASD and VSD repair surgery)

"Beth got heart block during her second surgery, in 1991, and then needed a pacemaker. It was hard to accept, but complications happen. Focus on the positive."

—Kathy Grampovnik, mom to Beth (aortic stenosis, subvalvular aortic stenosis, surgical heart block with a pacemaker)

Catheterization

What is cardiac catheterization?

Dr. Latson: Cardiac catheterization is a test in which a catheter—a very skinny, hollow tube—is inserted in a blood vessel and then moved into the heart. In children, catheters are most often inserted into the blood vessels in the groin. Sometimes catheters are inserted into vessels in the neck, arm, or other areas.

Are there specialized centers for catheterization?

Dr. O'Laughlin: While there are no approval or certification mechanisms for "specialized" centers for pediatric cardiac catheterization, there are certain hospitals or physicians who have particular interest and expertise in this type of catheterization. These centers are located throughout the United States and Canada and generally would be within reach of most patients. When selecting a pediatric catheterization center, ask questions about the experience of the physician, including specific number of procedures performed.

What do they look for or measure in a cardiac catheterization?

Dr. Latson: A cardiac catheterization is the only accurate way to measure pressures in all of the different chambers and blood vessels of the heart. During the catheterization, blood samples are usually obtained to measure the amount of oxygen in the blood in different chambers of the heart. It's possible to estimate how much blood is flowing to different areas of the heart with this information. In addition, a liquid known as "contrast" or "dye" can be injected through the catheter into a blood vessel or heart chamber. This dye shows up on X ray so that you can see details of the vessel or heart chamber.

What is the difference between diagnostic catheterization and therapeutic catheterization?

Dr. Latson: Diagnostic catheterization is done to obtain information. This information may be necessary to decide whether surgery or medications are needed. Therapeutic catheterization is done to change something inside the heart. In some patients, special catheters are used to open valves that are too tight, close abnormal blood vessels, or close some holes inside the heart.

What determines whether a child needs a catheterization?

Dr. Latson: Because there is a small risk to a cardiac catheterization, the procedure is done only if it is the safest of all the alternatives. A diagnostic catheterization is most often needed to accurately measure pressures in certain chambers of the heart or to outline fine details of certain types of heart defects. These details may be critical to the planning for a surgical procedure. A therapeutic catheterization is done only if there is a defect that is causing or could cause a significant problem. In each case, a decision must be made about whether a therapeutic catheterization is safer and better than a surgical procedure.

Can certain defects be repaired by catheterization?

Dr. Latson: Certain defects can be repaired very well by therapeutic catheterization procedures. There are excellent devices available to close some types of abnormal blood vessels. Special "balloon catheters" are used to open certain types of valves that are too tight or to enlarge narrowed areas in some blood vessels. In a few centers, very specialized devices to close certain types of holes in the heart also are available.

Who does the catheterization? Is it my cardiologist? What should his or her qualifications be?

Dr. Latson: Cardiac catheterization for pediatric patients with congenital heart defects should be done only by a qualified and experienced pediatric cardiologist. The pediatric cardiologist should have had special training in cardiac catheterization and should be doing cardiac catheterizations frequently.

Why can't my child eat before the catheterization?

Dr. Latson: You child shouldn't eat before a catheterization because he or she will likely be given some medications during the procedure that may cause nausea in some patients. Since your child may be sleepy for the catheterization, it could be dangerous if he or she vomits a large amount of material. It's safest if the stomach is empty before the catheterization is done.

How long does a catheterization take?

Dr. Latson: The time needed to do a catheterization depends on how complicated the procedure is. A diagnostic catheterization for a relatively simple heart defect may take only an hour or so. If the heart defect is more complicated or if several therapies or interventions need to be done, the catheterization can take six hours or more.

Does it involve general anesthesia? Will my child be sedated or awake?

Dr. Latson: Surprisingly, the catheter moving around inside the heart isn't painful. Children experience some pain when a local anesthetic—numbing medicine—is injected in the skin over the blood vessels where the catheters are inserted. Children must remain very still throughout the catheterization, so they're often given a sedative medication so they can sleep quietly throughout the procedure. If there is any concern about how well the child will breathe with heavy sedation, then it's safer to use general anesthesia.

What's the difference between sedation and general anesthesia?

Dr. Latson: When a child is sedated, he or she is simply sleeping quietly. Anything that causes very much pain will cause the child to wake up. General anesthesia is a much deeper level of sedation. When patients are under general anesthesia, they usually are so deeply asleep that they must have a machine to help them breathe.

Are there any side effects or risks with sedation and anesthesia?

Dr. O'Laughlin: There are risks from sedation in the cardiac catheterization laboratory. These include:

- Allergic or other reactions to the medicines used
- Oversedation leading to inadequate breathing
- Postcatheterization vomiting or drowsiness
- Low or high blood pressure
- Lack of oxygen
- Cyanotic (blue) spells
- Brain injury or damage, which might be permanent
- Death

The physicians and nurses in the catheterization laboratory are prepared to treat any reversible side effect from the sedation and to assist the patient with breathing as needed. All of these side effects are uncommon. In the judgment of the cardiologists recommending and performing the procedure, the risks of side effects combined with the risks of the procedure are outweighed by the risks of not performing the catheterization or of performing the catheterization without the sedation.

Specific risks from general anesthesia include all of the risks noted for general sedation and others. General anesthesia risks and other information should be obtained from the anesthesiologist who will do that part of the procedure.

Will my child be in pain during the catheterization?

Dr. Latson: Children should not be in pain during the catheterization. The only parts that cause significant discomfort are numbing of the skin where the catheters are inserted (this usually stings for about two minutes) and holding pressure over the blood vessel when the catheter is removed. If the catheterization procedure is long, then patients have difficulty holding still. They may experience some soreness in the back or shoulders from lying on a flat table.

Will my child have to spend the night at the hospital for a cardiac catheterization? Are there any situations in which my child would need to spend more than one night in the hospital?

Dr. Latson: Policies regarding how long a pediatric patient should stay in the hospital vary from institution to institution. In most centers that perform a lot of pediatric catheterizations, many of the procedures are done without an overnight hospital stay. Patients must be watched for several hours after a catheterization to be certain they are fully awake from the sedation or anesthesia and to be certain that there is no bleeding from the vessels where the catheters were inserted. If a therapeutic catheterization is done, then the child may need to stay in the hospital overnight to be certain that the therapy didn't change things too dramatically. It is rare that children are kept in the hospital for more than one night for a catheterization procedure. However, if a complication (such as a fever) occurs, then a longer stay in the hospital may be necessary.

"The night after his cath, we decided to let him stay in the hospital overnight. Even though we would have been in a hotel room nearby, it would've been hard to determine how worried I should be. It was reassuring to be there with the nurses. He couldn't eat much—just Jell-O and clear liquids. He had a rough night. He was very uncomfortable with the bandages and feeling lousy from the anesthesia. If I had gone to the hotel, I probably would have wound up going back to the hospital just to be reassured."

—*Robin Yankow, mom to Eddie (aortic stenosis, enlarged aortic root)*

What are the risks with cardiac catheterization?

Dr. Latson: There are always some risks involved when a catheter is placed inside the heart. The five major risks are:

1. The possibility of causing damage to the blood vessels where catheters are inserted. The blood vessels could be torn, there could be some bleeding from the vessels, or the vessels could become narrowed or occluded.

2. There is a possibility of causing some irregular rhythms when a catheter is moved inside the heart. If the heart beats too fast (tachycardia), it may be necessary to give some medications or even a shock. Rarely, a catheter can cause significant slowing of the heart rate that could possibly require a pacemaker.

3. There is a very small possibility that a catheter could perforate a wall of the heart or a blood vessel. This could require emergency surgery to repair.

4. There is a small chance that a clot or air bubble could form on a catheter. If this clot or air bubble comes loose, it could potentially block a small blood vessel in the lungs or even in the brain.

5. If a device is being placed in a therapeutic catheterization, then there is a small possibility that the device could move away from where it's supposed to be. This might require that the device be grabbed with another type of catheter and removed or might even require surgery to remove it.

How common are these risks?

Dr. Latson: The overall chance of a complication from cardiac catheterization is less than 1 percent. Certain patients may be at higher risk. Patients who are very young, very sick, or very cyanotic (blue babies) may be at higher risk for one or more complications. The complication rate for a therapeutic catheterization is generally higher than the rate for a single diagnostic catheterization.

How will my child feel after his catheterization?

Dr. O'Laughlin: As noted, your child may feel drowsy and unsteady after the procedure. His or her legs or other sites of catheter placement may be sore, and there may be some (or even a lot) of bruising at or near those sites. The child may have nausea or vomiting. For that reason, it is often suggested that the patient drink some clear liquid prior to trying formula, milk, or other foods. Sometimes the sites where the catheters were placed bleed through the dressing or bandage. (If that occurs, direct pressure with another gauze or a towel for five to ten minutes will likely stop the bleeding.) Rarely, there is some blood in the urine for a short time. The child may remember parts of the catheterization, particularly the injections of local anesthetic in the spots where the catheters will be introduced, or the needles themselves. Hallucinations occur rarely, and typically are short in duration if they happen.

Are there special things I need to do after the catheterization? Anything I need to look out for?

Dr. O'Laughlin: After cardiac catheterization, a patient may feel groggy or unsteady and may experience nausea or vomiting. The child should be encouraged to rest in bed the day of cardiac catheterization and should be told to expect these feelings, which occur when sedation or anesthesia wears off. The child should remain in bed reasonably immobile for two to six hours, depending on instructions from the physicians or nurses. This desire for quiet should be balanced against any discomfort or insecurity infants might feel not being allowed to move. Often they may be picked up and fed or otherwise comforted. Occasionally they will have a long board or boards on their legs to keep them from moving the legs and stirring up bleeding. If the bandages begin to ooze or bleed, direct pressure with a gauze pad or a washcloth will often stop the bleeding in a few minutes. The nurse or doctor should be notified of bleeding. We also recommend against soaking the catheter sites in water for about forty-eight hours after the procedure.

"We were told that Eddie shouldn't take a bath after his cath. This actually worked out well, as we got him into taking showers."
—*Robin Yankow, mom to Eddie (aortic stenosis, enlarged aortic root)*

How long is the recovery?

Dr. Latson: The recovery from a catheterization is usually fairly quick. Patients must wake up from any sedation or anesthesia they were given during the procedure. It may take several hours for the drugs to wear off completely. The leg where catheters are inserted may be sore for several days. There commonly is a small bruise. The soreness usually is not severe, and most children are able to return to normal activities within one or two days after the catheterization procedure.

Types of Catheterization Procedures

What is a blade septostomy? When is it used?

Dr. O'Laughlin: A blade septostomy is a heart catheterization technique for making or enlarging a hole in the wall between the upper chambers of the heart, or the atrial septum. To perform a blade septostomy, the cardiologist first maneuvers a sheath or tube across the heart wall, either

by going through a small natural hole or by poking through the atrial septum with a long needle into the left chamber (atrium). Through that sheath
a special catheter with a recessed blade is passed into the left atrium; then
the blade is exposed and the entire catheter and sheath apparatus is drawn
back to the right, cutting the tissue in the wall and enlarging the communication. The process is repeated a number of times to ensure a good-sized
hole in the wall between the upper chambers. It is usually followed by a
balloon septostomy or balloon dilatation of the wall to create the final
opening. In recent years the blade septostomy has been used less and balloon dilatation of the heart wall used more.

What is a balloon catheter? When is it used?

Dr. O'Laughlin: The typical balloon catheter is a long tube onto the tip
of which is built a sausage-shaped balloon. Initially, the balloon is deflated
and wrapped snugly around the end of the catheter. When the balloon is in
place across a narrow part of the heart (such as a valve), it's inflated. It then
stretches or tears the valve, artery, or vein. The tube or catheter itself can
be placed over a wire during a heart catheterization, making it easier to get
into position. When the physician sees that the length of the balloon strad-
dles the area to be enlarged, he or she then inflates the balloon.

A balloon catheter is used when you need to dilate or enlarge a cardiovascular structure. The structure may be a valve, a vessel, a conduit, or
another structure. The balloon enlargement procedure may delay or eliminate the need for surgery in some cases.

What is pulmonary valvuloplasty? When is it used?

Dr. O'Laughlin: Pulmonary valvuloplasty is the cardiac catheterization
procedure of balloon dilatation of the pulmonary valve, the valve leading
from the right ventricle (pumping chamber) to the pulmonary artery (lung
artery). The procedure is performed as described above (see the material
on the balloon catheter) and often results in partial or complete relief of
blockage at the valve level.

The procedure is used when there is a blockage or narrowing at the
level of the pulmonary valve. This is done whenever the level of obstruction is moderate or severe, as judged by the catheterizing physician.

What is a cineangiogram? When is it used?

Dr. O'Laughlin: A cineangiogram is an X-ray movie of a heart chamber
or blood vessel. It is made by injection of contrast material, a liquid that
shows up on X ray, into the blood in the chamber or vessel of interest. As
the heart beats, the fluid moves with the blood, showing the details of the

anatomy. It is used as part of most heart catheterizations, to investigate the status of the patient's heart and blood vessels.

What is angiocardiography? When is it used?

Dr. O'Laughlin: Angiocardiography is a general term for taking pictures of the heart and blood vessels. It is done by means of cineangiograms, as detailed in the previous answer.

What is a coil procedure for a PDA? Is it effective?

Dr. O'Laughlin: A coil procedure for a patent ductus arteriosus (PDA) is a cardiac catheterization procedure in which a stainless steel coil with fiber threads attached to it is permanently implanted in the abnormal vessel (the PDA) to close it. This is done as part of a heart catheterization and in most cases will eliminate the PDA without the need for surgery. In the procedure, a catheter or tube is maneuvered from the leg to and across the abnormal vessel under X-ray guidance. Then a small coil is inserted (in a straightened shape) into the catheter and pushed up until it comes out of the end of the catheter and begins to resume its coil shape. Part of the coil is placed on the lung artery side of the PDA, and then the coil wire is brought back to the aortic side of the PDA and pushed the rest of the way out. By straddling the PDA and placing the bulk of metal and fabric across the vessel, the coil makes a clot form and closes the PDA from the inside. Occasionally more than one coil is required to close the PDA completely.

The coil procedure is very effective overall in closing PDAs, and it eliminates the need for surgery in more than 90 percent of patients in whom it is used. Sometimes there is a small leak after the coil is placed, but often it closes in days to weeks. With continued closure over time and a rare second procedure, the success rises to more than 95 percent. It is applicable in most centers only for tiny, small, or medium-sized PDAs rather than large ones.

Can an ASD be closed by catheterization? How effective is this?

Dr. O'Laughlin: Small to moderate-sized secundum atrial septal defects have been closed successfully over the years with a variety of catheter-delivered devices. Currently none of those devices is approved for use in the United States. There are some devices that have been undergoing study in approved Food and Drug Administration protocols. In these studies and others taking place in Europe and other places, there appears to be approximately a 92 to 95 percent chance of procedural success. Procedural success means that the device is implanted in or across the atrial septal defect at the time of catheterization. Some of the "successful" patients have leftover leaks around the implanted devices, but many of those leaks appear to close with time. These devices may be of use in patients who have a normal tiny atrial communication called a patent foramen ovale or PFO and who have had a stroke. It appears reasonable for a patient or parents to inquire about the status of these types of devices if surgery is recommended for a small or moderate-sized secundum atrial septal defect or patent foramen ovale.

My child has a closed valve, and they want to do a catheterization. Is this okay?

Dr. O'Laughlin: A number of congenital heart diseases include a narrow or obstructed valve. Usually cardiac catheterization is reasonable in these conditions. Often balloon dilatation of the closed valve is possible at the time of the catheterization (see material on the balloon catheter and pulmonary valve dilatation earlier in this chapter). In other cases the cardiac catheterization is performed in preparation for or to follow up on results of surgery. In mild cases of blockage, or in cases in which surgery alone is the correct treatment, catheterization may not be necessary.

ZACK'S STORY
As told by his mom, Ilene Weiss

Our son Zack was born with a VSD. We found out when he was one week old. I was hysterical. He was my firstborn, and he had a problem with his heart. We went to a cardiologist who assured us that he had a perfectly normal hole, that a lot of babies were born with this condition, and that it probably would close in time. We began what was a series of yearly visits to the cardiologists to keep track of his condition.

As he approached the age of five or six, we were told that while the VSD was not getting bigger in relation to the size of his growing heart, it would probably never close. We were told not to worry. Many people live normal, active lives with VSDs.

In the fall of 1996 we went for our usual checkup. I expected to hear the same "don't worry, Mrs. Weiss, the hole isn't getting any smaller but everything is okay" line from our doctor. Instead, he told us that he saw a leakage of sorts in Zack's aortic valve and wanted to keep a closer eye on him. Could we come back in six months? I believe I didn't panic at that time only because I probably didn't fully understand or didn't want to understand what he was saying.

We went for a second opinion at another medical center. The cardiologist there confirmed what the first one had said. She, too, recommended that we come back in six months. We did—there was little or no change, so again I left feeling okay.

On November 24, 1997, we went for our routine yearly visit. The usual echo was done. Afterward, with our son (now nine) in the consultation room with us, the cardiologist told us that she felt there was more aortic leakage than before. There was the potential of open-heart surgery, but before we thought about anything she wanted to do a cardiac catheterization just to get a closer look. At that moment two things happened. I looked at my son and realized he was white as a ghost. He obviously was not old enough or mature enough to hear about a tube that was going to invade his body. And I knew, even though no one had said so, that he was going to have to have open-heart surgery.

My husband, my son, and I left the doctor's office. We were all in a state of shock. After the doctor's visit, my husband and I had planned to go back to work and take Zack to school. We all cried and went to the movies instead. Zack cried because he was scared about this tube that was going to invade his body. We cried because we knew our son was going to be cut open. I was afraid he was going to die.

The doctor called later that evening to apologize for talking in front of Zack. She thought he was old enough to handle it. I was disappointed that she didn't ask me first. Zack was very scared. We tried to answer all his questions the best we could. He was most afraid of the IV that would be put into his arm to sedate him. We tried to calm his fears over the course of a few days—to no avail. The only thing that calmed him down was knowing we were going for a second opinion and that the procedure was still far off.

In early December, after doing some research on doctors, we went for another opinion to confirm the necessity of a catheterization.

The doctor examined Zack, had an echo done, and then it was time to talk. We spent an hour with him. Zack waited outside with his grandfather. We were not going to make that same mistake again.

The doctor told us that there was no point in putting Zack through a catheterization. Between what he heard and saw on the echo, it was very clear that Zack's problems had to be fixed—the open-heart surgery was confirmed. The questions was when. I started going over the edge, afraid that Zack was going to die.

We met up with Zack and his grandfather. We told him no catheterization for him. He was thrilled. We didn't tell him about the impending surgery, since we had no idea when it would take place. We didn't want him to be burdened with it for too long.

We went home. I was numb. When do we do the surgery? During the summer? Now? In the spring? We finally decided since the recuperation was two months we didn't want to mess up Zack's summer or his spring. We spoke to his teacher, who told us not to worry, Zack was bright and was entitled to a tutor when he was ready. We decided to do the surgery as soon as possible. Part of our decision not to wait was selfish—Zack's dad and I wanted it over as soon as possible.

The call came at 9:00 P.M. on December 30, 1997. Zack's cardiologist told us he had looked at the surgeon's schedule. How was January 28? I almost fainted.

So began the longest month of our lives. How and when do we tell Zack?

We couldn't sleep, I barely ate, I went on antidepressants—I was afraid Zack was going to die. When people in my office began finding out and they would come over and try to comfort me, I couldn't talk about it—I began to cry. I asked people not to mention it to me—I could not deal with it. Now I began to be afraid that I would break down when I spoke to Zack. They say all a child has to do is look in your eyes and he or she knows whether to be afraid.

We began the process of trying to figure out how to tell him. We knew we weren't going to tell him too far in advance. About two weeks before the surgery, we started seeing Child Life specialists at Babies' Hospital. After discussing how Zack reacted to the prospect of a catheterization, the Child Life specialist agreed we should give him some time but not as little as we were going to. The operation was on a Wednesday. We were going to tell him Friday. She thought he needed a week. We went home and talked about it. Did we want to deal with Zack knowing for a week?

Next, we went to see a psychiatrist with the cardiac unit. He also suggested that Zack needed a week to desensitize himself to the process and see the hospital.

Now, what about me? I saw a hypnotherapist who deals with cardiac patients. We talked, she gave me hypnotic suggestions, I practiced, and felt I could look Zack in the eye.

We were especially frustrated because we couldn't find anyone who had a nine-year-old who had gone through this and find out how they reacted. Most kids who have VSDs have them closed young. Zack also had a mild aortic insufficiency that made the surgery more risky.

The mothers I was put in touch with through support groups were very caring, but their kids were so much more critical than Zack it was hard for me to relate to what they were going through—our situations were very different.

On January 21, 1998, one week before the operation, we told Zack. We told him that the doctor had just called and determined the surgery was necessary and—Guess what?—the surgeon we wanted had an opening the following week.

Of course, Zack got hysterical—but only briefly. How could we make the surgery so soon? We explained that we didn't want to mess up the warm months, but certainly if he was not ready, we could wait. He thought about it and then told us he guessed it really didn't matter when we told him and when the surgery was—he would still be afraid. We told him we would all get through this together. He asked minimal surgery questions that night. I came through with flying colors. His biggest concern was the IV. Could he be put to sleep with a mask? We told him we would see what we could do. The following day we took him to see my hypnotherapist. She spoke with him and gave him some relaxation techniques that would hopefully get him through his tension. He went home and went to school. His teacher had been warned and was the best.

Friday, we took him to Child Life. They showed him everything they could and explained things. When they got to the IV part, Zack almost fainted. He insisted no one was putting an IV in his arm while he was awake. Other than that, they were terrific.

Monday, we went for preop testing and more hospital touring. Everyone was wonderful. The doctor said he would see what he could do about a mask for surgery to put him under. We took one home to practice.

Tuesday, we all went about our regular business, which was the best way we could deal with things. Zack went to school. We went to work. I was out of my mind.

Wednesday—January 28—surgery day. We arrived at the hospital at 8:00 A.M. for 10:00 A.M. surgery. An emergency transplant was happening, forcing us to spend the next five hours trying to entertain ourselves. Just as we were feeling the surgery might be postponed (the last thing we wanted!), we got the call to go to preop. Zack panicked. We couldn't get him from the tenth to the fourth floor. It took us half an hour to coax him down. We were promised something to relax him. He drank it. They told him it might make him sleepy and suggested he lie down. He wouldn't because he knew once he lay down on the gurney, surgery was imminent. He passed out five minutes later in a chair. Thank God we didn't have to walk him into the OR and wait until he was sedated. I cried—a lot from relief that it was finally here but mostly because I was afraid I would never see my son again.

We passed the time with family and friends. At 6:15 P.M. the surgeon arrived in the ICU waiting room. The surgery was over and it was a success. We would be able to see Zack in a few minutes.

I was expecting the worst. People had told me he would be green, bloated, look horrible. Zack looked terrific. We stayed for a while and then left, since he was heavily sedated and we knew we would need our strength for the days ahead.

When we returned Thursday at 5:00 A.M. the nurse told us Zack had been up most of the night but wasn't afraid to be there. He knew what was happening—his mom and dad had explained it all to him—he wrote to the nurse. She told us we should be very proud—we had prepared him well!

ZACK'S STORY
By Zachary Weiss, age ten

When my mom and dad told me about the operation I was mad. Why did it have to happen to me?

During the days leading up to the surgery, I tried not to think about the operation. School took my mind off of it. When I tried to go to sleep, it was hard. Thinking about having it done was so out of this world. You think it can't happen to you then—boom—it happens.

The day of the operation was boring. I had to wait five hours for the surgery. The nurses were very nice. They gave me things to do and let me go to the playroom.

You don't know what will happen next. Then they call your name. I was so scared. I wouldn't go to the operating room.

I didn't want to know what would happen next. I wouldn't lie down on the stretcher because I knew the next thing was the operation. They gave me a cocktail and I drifted off.

When I woke up my mom and dad were there. I was tied down, had IVs, couldn't talk, drink, eat—my mouth was dry.

My chest was so sore I couldn't feel it.

Every time they cleaned my ventilator out it made me cough and it really hurt—but luckily it didn't last very long.

The food was terrible. My chest hurt. I didn't want to use the pain management because it made me itch.

My mom told me if I didn't get up and start clearing my lungs, the doctors would clean them out with a needle.

They got you up early in the morning for blood tests. My arterial line hurt when it came out.

The day I got out of the hospital it was hard walking to the car. Then it was hard sitting in the car.

I was starving.

I was home.

CHAPTER 6

THE HOSPITAL STAY

Betsy Adler, M.S.N., R.N., C.P.N.P.   Dennis Sklenar, C.S.W.
Peter B. Manning, M.D.   Gil Wernovsky, M.D.
Kenneth O. Schowengerdt, Jr., M.D.   Lisa Wispé, M.S.N., R.N., C.P.N.P.
Howard Zucker, M.D., J.D.

THIS roller-coaster ride that I described in chapter 3 can get wilder as you approach the day of surgery. It's something that was echoed many times by other parents we've talked to. Be prepared for it. You might expect it if your child were waiting for a heart transplant, but it happens to all of us, whatever the defect. Children get sick—the normal coughing, sneezing, aching head kind of sick—and surgery gets put off. Even doctors get sick, or go on vacation, and you have to plan around their schedules. Or you make it to surgery day and then an emergency comes in and your child's surgery is postponed hours or even a full day. (Always try to have your child's surgery scheduled as early as possible in the morning, so that if an emergency does come in, you're less likely to have to wait an entire day for a new surgery slot.) All of this takes an emotional toll, but at least if you know in advance things might not happen as planned, you'll be able to deal with it a little better.

We'd spent some time prepping for Max's hospital stay—mostly by having talks with our pediatric cardiologist and a Roanoke parent who had just gotten back from Duke. But when we got to the hospital, I wasn't really prepared for all the people who were suddenly part of our lives. Nurses, doctors, residents, interns.

We took our place in the surgical waiting room. I looked around at all of these people waiting to hear about their children. There was some comfort in knowing we weren't the only ones dealing with this, but there were a lot of other emotions, too. Guilt that our child's problem wasn't as serious as another's. Jealousy that another's child was less serious than ours. Fear that Max's condition could become more complex, like the child of the woman sitting next to me in the waiting room. Despite all of our preparation, no one prepared me for this.

We were somewhat in denial. Max's diagnosis was tetralogy of Fallot—one of the most common and treatable forms of CHD. He would be repaired and we would go about normal life. He just wouldn't be allowed to play football or wrestle in high school. His problem wasn't serious. At least that's what we kept telling ourselves. We'd deal with it and move on.

And for those of you with children who have much more severe or complex forms of CHD, tetralogy probably does seem relatively minor. The facts are, though, that any surgery is risky, and any CHD is, to one degree or another, a lifelong concern—facts we weren't completely ready to face.

Whether intending to or not, the doctors bolstered our denial, each one assuring us that TOF repair was "all in a day's work," that they do them all the time. What may seem a big deal to us is business-as-usual to them.

We wanted to believe them, and accordingly refused to let any of our family travel to North Carolina to be with us. A rallying of the troops would make this ordeal seem too serious. We didn't want people fussing over us or worrying about us (as if they weren't doing that long distance). We told them to save their money and their vacation time and visit us at home, when everything was over. Nurses and doctors talked to us about the wires and tubes that Max would be hooked up to after surgery. They told us he'd be swollen and puffy. And they took us on a tour of the PICU before Max took his place there.

Just about every CHD parent we've talked to while writing this book told us how helpful it was or would have been to see pictures of kids in the PICU, so we encourage you to find them on the Internet. Personally, I hated touring the PICU, but I am definitely in the minority. I didn't want to see other people's helpless children, since I knew I'd have to face my own soon enough. And when the time came, despite the fact that Max looked very different from his usual self lying there—face puffy, tubes and wires everywhere—he was still my baby and I was just glad to be back at his side.

The greatest piece of advice I can give anyone who will have a child in the PICU is to befriend the incredible nurses who keep watch over your child. Recognize that each one is a human being and that they don't all do their job the same way. I desperately wanted to hold Max. That loss of physical contact with him was the most difficult part of his being in the PICU. One nurse I asked was worried about the tubes and wires, and kept putting me off. Maybe the next day, she would say. But when I asked the nurses on different shifts, some allowed it, some didn't. Some probably would have let me hold him a day earlier if I hadn't assumed that what went for one nurse went for all.

Pumping my breast milk, which is not my most favorite thing in the world, also helped me get through that period. It was the one thing, aside from sitting bedside, that I could really do for Max. It made me feel productive. And boy, was I. When we left the hospital, I was presented with an embarrassingly large tray full of the bottles of milk I had collected.

I am sure you have many concerns about your hospital stay. Hospitals can be scary, intimidating places, particularly on your first visit. They are full of all sorts of people, machines, and procedures that you are totally unfamiliar with. We have put together some information to help prepare you for this visit. Because hospital policies vary, it's impossible to address many specific issues. We have tried to give you the tools to ask the right questions of your hospital before your child is admitted. It will probably be helpful to take this book with you so that if you have any questions during your child's stay you can have an instant reference.

Gerri

An Overview of the Hospital Stay (by Gil Wernovsky, M.D.)

Preparing your child (and family) for an inpatient stay is one of the most important ways you can contribute to your child's recovery. Knowing what to expect *before* surgery will help to ease the psychological stress as well as speed recovery. It is beyond the scope of this chapter to provide *all* necessary information specific for you and your child, because:

1. hospital policies and guidelines vary, and
2. the recovery process is different for
    a. different operations
    b. children of different ages
    c. medical condition of the child going into surgery

The following are some general suggestions. Always consult your child's primary care team (pediatrician, cardiologist, and surgeon) for specific details.

The Preoperative Period

It's helpful to ask questions of your child's care team *before* the scheduled surgery. A preoperative visit with your child's surgeon and cardiologist—a few weeks before the procedure, if possible—will allow time to address questions that come up. If your child is younger than a teenager or so, consider making this visit *without* your child, to allow for your full attention. Bring a list of questions with you, to be sure everything is answered to your satisfaction before the end of your visit. It's a good idea to keep a journal or notebook, to write down your questions before (or after) your visit, and to refresh your memory at a later date. This is a stressful time, and you shouldn't expect to remember everything in one sitting.

As a general guideline, the amount of time a child needs to cope with the prospect of surgery increases with the age of the child. A child will need about one day of "preparation" for each year of age—a three-year-old may only need a few days, while a preadolescent may need a week or more. You will be the best judge of your own child's psychological needs, but *always* give your child preparation time before surgery. Don't tell your child on the day of pretesting that she is going to stay in the hospital. Consult your pediatrician, family physician, and cardiac team as you are deciding when to tell her. It's usually a good idea to bring a favorite toy, pillowcase, or stuffed animal along with your child. Check with your hospital for guidelines and suggestions. Many hospitals have Child Life or "play therapy" specialists whom you may contact before the hospitalization for specific instructions, guidelines, and preoperative teaching.

The Physical Facility

After heart surgery, most children will stay in a special unit of the hospital called an intensive care unit (ICU). In many hospitals, newborns will be in an area designated as the neonatal intensive care unit, commonly referred to as NICU (pronounced nick-U), and other babies and children will be placed in an area called the pediatric intensive care unit or PICU (pronounced pick-U). These units are specially equipped to deal with the infant or child returning from the operating room (OR), and are designed to contain a great deal of monitoring equipment, machines, and personnel. Some hospitals have dedicated areas of a general ICU, or even an entirely separate ICU specifically for children recovering from heart surgery. Inside the ICU, you'll hear alarms and unfamiliar noises; the staff is specially trained to respond to these alarms.

Some questions you should ask include:

- Where will my child go before surgery?
- Will I be able to accompany my child into the OR before he or she is sedated?
- Where will I wait during surgery?

- Will my child go to a recovery room, stepdown area, or ICU after surgery?
- Will there be other children my child's age and/or other children with heart problems there?
- After the ICU, where will my child recover until hospital discharge?

The Personnel

While in the ICU, your child will have a specific group of nurses and physicians specially trained in monitoring and evaluating your child's recovery. The amount of nursing coverage in an ICU is called the "nurse-patient ratio"; it is generally 1:1 immediately after surgery, and as your child recovers will gradually move to 1:2 (one nurse for two patients) and then 1:3 or more as he or she gets ready for hospital discharge.

A group of specially trained physicians will work together with the nursing staff to provide care immediately after surgery. This will include your child's surgeon and some or all of the following:

- *Anesthesiologists* (physicians trained in artificial breathing [respirators], and the use of medications to allow for pain-free and memory-free surgery)
- *Intensivists* (physicians trained to care for critically ill patients, sometimes with additional training in anesthesia)
- *Cardiologists* (heart specialists)
- *Neonatologists* (physicians trained in newborn medicine)
- Various other specialists (e.g., in infectious diseases, gastroenterology, genetics, neurology, etc.) may be called in for consultation as necessary

If you're at a teaching hospital, "physicians in training"—medical students, interns, residents, and fellows—also will care for your child. This might get confusing, so don't hesitate to ask who is who and what role they are playing in your child's care.

Finally, additional personnel will complete the care team, including respiratory therapists, Child Life specialists, pharmacists, clergy, and social workers.

Some specific questions to ask include:

- What is the composition of the care team in the ICU and on the floor?
- What is the role of my child's surgeon, cardiologist, and the rest of the team?

- Who is in charge of my child's care?
- Are there physicians in training who will assist my child's care team and be able to answer my questions?
- When will I meet with the surgeon and my child's care team after surgery?
- How will I be updated on my child's progress after surgery?
- Who will keep me informed?
- Who will notify my child's pediatrician or family physician of my child's operation?

Hospital Guidelines and Policies

Each hospital, ICU, and ward has different guidelines and policies that you should know before your child undergoes surgery. Questions you could ask are:

- What are the visitation guidelines after surgery in the ICU?
- Can siblings visit?
- Who will receive information after surgery?
- Can my relatives call for updates?
- What facilities are available for sleep at night?
- May I sleep next to my child in the ICU and/or ward?
- Is there a laundry facility available? Cash machine? Breast pump?
- May I donate blood for my child?

Each day, physicians, nurses, and other personnel will review your child's progress and plan her care. This process—called "rounds"—is extremely important in the transfer of information from caregiver to caregiver. It also serves as a teaching exercise in hospitals with physicians in training. You should ask about your hospital's policies on parents' attendance during rounds. Hospitals vary greatly in this regard. Sometimes parents will be asked to leave during rounds or the nursing report at shift change, because confidential information may be discussed about other patients in the ICU. It is important to understand that there are no "secrets" about your child discussed during these rounds and that you are fully entitled to up-to-the-minute information. It is sometimes more efficient for the care team to make rounds in your absence. If this is the case, be sure you receive a complete summary of the care plan from your child's nurse and/or physician at the completion of rounds.

In addition, you may be asked to leave the ICU if the staff is busy concentrating on the care of your child or one in her vicinity, or when a child is having a procedure or has just returned from the operating room.

The Procedure

The enormous variability of surgical procedures for congenital heart disease precludes giving specific information in this chapter. In general, the past decade has witnessed tremendous advances in the management of congenital heart disease. Corrective procedures are performed more frequently in younger and younger children. In addition to the details of the surgical procedure, its risks, and expected results, specific questions to ask your care team may include:

- How long is my child likely to be in the hospital?
- Is a blood transfusion likely?
- Will the heart/lung machine be necessary ("open-heart" surgery)?
- Will my child be on medications at discharge?
- How will my child's pain be managed postoperatively?

Lines, Tubes, and What Are All of These Machines?

After open-heart surgery, children are usually connected in various ways to wires, tubes, and machines, each of which has a specific job to ensure your child's recovery. Each makes a special noise or alarm to notify the care team of a change. Remember, most alarms don't signal a problem, just a change from the previous values. The nurses and physicians will recognize these changes and react appropriately.

Immediately after surgery, your child still will have residual effects of anesthesia and may not be strong or awake enough to breathe on her own. There will be a tube running (either through her nose or mouth) directly into her breathing tube (trachea) to allow a machine (respirator or ventilator) to do the work of breathing until she's fully awake and has regained her strength. After more complex types of surgery, especially in young infants, continuous intravenous medications may be administered to rest the heart and lungs and relieve pain. In these cases the breathing muscles may be weak enough or the child sleepy enough to extend the period of time on the ventilator by a few days or longer.

Your child will get fluid, nutrition, pain medications, antibiotics, and heart medications through intravenous lines (catheters) inserted into a large vein in the neck, groin, or directly through the chest into the heart chambers. Additionally, larger tubes are often necessary under the skin into the chest (chest tubes) to drain any small amounts of blood or fluid that might otherwise build up. Especially if the heart/lung machine is used (open-heart surgery), children may appear puffy and swollen. To help reduce this swelling, extra fluid may be expelled through the urine with medication (diuretics) or from the abdomen through catheters (peritoneal dialysis). All of these tubes, catheters, wires, and the temporary change in your child's appearance may be quite frightening at first. We recommend a preoperative tour to prepare you and your family for these events.

TIPS FOR THE HOSPITAL STAY

"As a parent, you have to get some rest when you can (it's very hard to do), but you have to, and you have to eat! If you don't eat and you get weak and sick, it's not going to help your child because you won't be able to go into the hospital room with your child because you're sick, and they *can't* get sick after surgery."

—*Victoria Drawant, mom to Crystal (anomalous left coronary, mitral valve prolapse with regurgitation, and pulmonary stenosis)*

"Realistically, parents will have a hard time taking care of themselves during this time. You have to keep eating sensibly, and take something with you to occupy your time. If there is a sibling at home, you're torn apart there because they miss you and want everyone home again at the same time. Spouses have to take turns staying at the hospital and then going home to other children. This is hard because while you're away (from the hospital) you're worried about changes, and while you're at the hospital you're worried about the children at home."

—*Sharon Popp, mom to Ben (pulmonary atresia with VSD and transposition of the aorta)*

"We had bought special books and a special easel to use in bed and favorite animals/toys. The Mylar balloons were great, too. Take your camera—use it and keep a journal of your whole experience."

—*Sheryl Lamb, mom to Heather (double outlet right ventricle, hypoplastic right upper chamber, transposition, subvalvular pulmonary stenosis, bilateral superior vena cava with interrupted inferior vena cava, common ventricle)*

"We had a lot of relatives waiting with us during surgery. It's hard to listen to everyday conversation and watch people play cards while your child is lying in the OR with his chest cracked open. I chose to distance myself some by going for walks and sitting in the chapel. Be glad they're there for you and for your child, but don't feel like you have to entertain them. Take care of yourself and your own needs at the time."

—*Susie DeLoach, mom to Joey (HLHS)*

"Make a list of questions to ask when the surgeon or cardiologist comes by—they're usually not there long and you can get distracted once they're there."
—*Anne Linne, mom to Kevin* (*transposition of the great vessels*)

"Don't tell your child that he will be in the hospital only a certain amount of days, because complications can arise."
—*Kathy Grampovnik, mom to Beth* (*aortic stenosis, subvalvular aortic stenosis, surgical heart block with a pacemaker*)

"In the hospital, listen to what the doctors tell you to look for to learn how to take care of your child yourself. The doctors and the nurses can't be there all the time to monitor them so you have to be able to do that for your child."
—*Pat Posada Klapper, mom to Alexandra* (*VSD*)

"Leaving the room and taking walks helped, especially in the first few days following surgery, when he was too drugged to miss me. Those first couple of nights were also when I went home to get some uninterrupted sleep. It was hard to leave Alex alone in the hospital, but I knew he was being given the best care and I was only in the way. As days went on and Alex improved, that's when he needed and wanted me to be there for him at every moment and I felt compelled to respond to his every cry now that I was able to soothe him. . . . Also, whenever someone comes to visit at the hospital, don't feel the need to play hostess. Let them sit with your child while you take a nap or step out for a breath of fresh air."
—*Sara Daniel, mom to Alex* (*tricuspid atresia, ASD, VSD*)

"We purchased a "special friend" (a stuffed Dalmatian puppy) to take to the hospital with us—he has accompanied our child on every subsequent visit to the hospital. Also, let them control whatever they can—what they eat, what they watch—they feel so overcontrolled at the hospital."
—*Joanne Baldauf, mom to Kenny* (*double inlet left ventricle with outflow chamber, transposition of the great vessels*)

"I found out that talking with the other mothers in the hospital unit helped me through."
—*Dawn Howie, mom to Travis* (*HLHS*)

"At least once or twice while your child is in the hospital go out for a nice dinner."
—*Lisa Kay Hartmann, mom to Jenna* (*tetralogy of Fallot with pulmonary atresia*)

"Keep in touch over the phone. When I was really stressed out (at the hospital) . . . updating people helped pass the time."

—Susan Wirth, mom to Julia (interrupted aortic arch, VSD, ASD)

"Find out what the staff expects of parents, find out what services are provided to you, and double-check that nurses get and pass on information between shifts."

—Stephen Slobodnik, dad to Laura (HLHS, coarctation of the aorta, AVSD)

"It helps to do as much as you can for them (i.e., combing their hair, rubbing moisturizer where you can, singing to them, etc.)"

—Diane and Trent Barilko, parents to Alexandra (double outlet right ventricle, pulmonary atresia with a VSD, discontinuous LPA, major aorta/pulmonary collateral arterials, pulmonary branch stenosis)

"If you're ready for a break from your visitors, tell them to leave you alone for a while."

—Deanna Smith, mom to Nicholas (HLHS)

"While in the NICU and PICU, I found it was helpful to read her chart and be part of what was going on, doing as much babycare as possible, and being informed about her medical care. And rocking, rocking, rocking my baby as much as possible."

—Laura Murphy, mom to Amanda (hypertrophic cardiomyopathy and Noonan's syndrome)

"Don't get hung up on your expected 'date of departure' from the hospital, because you never know what might delay it. Instead, focus on day-to-day improvements and learn to live without a schedule for a while."

—Gerri Freid Kramer, mom to Max (tetralogy of Fallot)

In the ICU

I'm afraid that my child will try to rip out his tubes or respirator. What can be done to prevent this?

Dr. Zucker: This is a common problem with children. Since these tubes are very important, we often give medications to keep children comfortable. Besides taking away the pain, these medications make the children sleepy. Sometimes we reach the maximum amount of medication we like to give and then we add soft restraints called no-no's (as in "No, no. Don't pull that tube out!"). These are soft, padded armboards that prevent the child from pulling at important tubes and wires.

What is a normal heart rate?

Dr. Zucker: Heart rates vary based on many factors, including age, level of arousal, fever, and medications. It's important that moms and dads not get fixed on a certain number. We usually use the following general guidelines:

Infants	120–140 bpm (beats per minute)
Toddlers	100–120 bpm
Children	80–100 bpm
Adolescents	60–80 bpm

Medications that help the heart squeeze often increase the heart rate by 20 to 30 percent. Every degree Celsius temperature rise above normal causes the body to get revved up by approximately 5 to 10 percent. Lastly, sometimes children need to have their hearts paced at a faster rate, even 50 percent higher than normal. We often look at heart rates not as a single number but over the course of a day.

"When I first saw him, he had just come out of surgery. He was bloated, discolored, and hooked up to so many tubes, I was afraid to touch him. The nurse told me that his heart rate went down when I got there. Hearing my voice comforted him."

—Carole Stoll, mom to Zachary
(VSD, subaortic stenosis, interrupted aortic arch)

What is a normal blood pressure?

Dr. Zucker: Blood pressure is much like heart rate, and dependent on the same factors. A good rule of thumb is to flip the heart rate guidelines to assess systolic (upper number) blood pressure:

Infants	60
Toddlers	80
Children	100
Adolescents	120

Blood pressure is comprised of two numbers: The systolic is the upper number and the diastolic is the lower number. As much as we look at the numbers independently, we also look at the difference between the two numbers, which is called the pulse pressure. Among other things, it reflects the fluid status of the baby, the functioning of one of the major valves of the heart, and whether there is any fluid surrounding the heart.

It seems as if there are a lot of bells and whistles going off. How do the nurses distinguish these?

Dr. Zucker: Just as a mom and a dad can distinguish their baby's cry from other children's cries, so nurses and doctors can identify specific bells and alarms as their cue to check a specific machine. The companies who make these machines work together to assure that two alarms from equipment that are often used together do not sound alike. The alarm setting can be adjusted and, therefore, sometimes the child's monitors will seem to be "communicating" more frequently than at other times. More often than not, the alarms are reminders that the IV fluids need to be replenished, the humidifier needs to be adjusted, or the temperature needs to be checked rather than actually signifying a medical problem.

Why does my child have abnormal heart rhythm after surgery? How is this treated?

Dr. Schowengerdt: Abnormal rhythms after heart surgery may occur for several reasons. Certain types of congenital heart disease may be associated with rhythm abnormalities, and the rigors of the heart/lung bypass machine may temporarily affect the heart muscle, making it more prone to abnormal rhythms. In addition, the incisions and stitches that may be required within the heart as part of the operation may cause an abnormal rhythm for a period of time. Certain medications used to stimulate the heart and aid its function after a major operation may also lower the threshold for the development of abnormal rhythms.

Abnormal rhythms occurring after heart surgery are often self-limited and may not necessarily require long-term therapy. Your child will be monitored closely in the intensive care unit after surgery so that these abnormal rhythms, if they occur, can be treated appropriately, often with medication.

EXPERIENCING ICU

"The first time you see your infant in ICU, it's overwhelming. Be prepared for a zillion wires and tubes. If possible, have a chair handy to sink into when you feel like you're going to faint. Look at pictures of other babies ahead of time if you can, to prepare you for what you are going to see (it's still not the same, because it's not *your* baby in the pictures)."

—*Sue Dove, mom to Scott (single ventricle)*

"Don't stare at the monitors; you'll drive yourself nuts. . . . Be aware of where the numbers should be, but don't get paranoid over every little alarm."

—*Susie DeLoach, mom to Joey (HLHS)*

"The chest tubes and IVs, monitors, and noise were scary and a lot to take at our first experience. The second surgery was a lot better because we knew what to expect."

—*Sheryl Lamb, mom to Heather (double outlet right ventricle,*
hypoplastic right upper chamber, transposition,
subvalvular pulmonary stenosis, bilateral superior vena cava with
interrupted inferior vena cava, common ventricle)

"When Kevin was three, he saw a picture of himself as a baby hooked up to a lot of IVs and a ventilator. He asked where the baby pictures were of his brother and sister with their tubes."

—*Anne Linne, mom to Kevin (transposition of the great vessels)*

"I wasn't prepared for all the wires, monitors, and tubes that were hooked up to him after surgery. Only being a little over three pounds for the surgery, all the equipment hooked up to him were astonishing. . . . I was amazed, though, that most of them were removed within a day or two after the surgery and how small the scar was."

—*Dawn Howie, mom to Travis (HLHS)*

What is a pulse oximeter? Will it hurt my child?

Dr. Zucker: A pulse oximeter is used to measure the oxygen level in your child's blood. It looks like a small red light and is not painful or even hot to the touch. When it's placed on a finger or a toe, it transmits heart rate and oxygen level to a machine. It is extremely sensitive to changes and is an excellent predictor of whether additional oxygen being provided to your son or daughter needs to be increased or decreased. Sometimes the overhead light in the room can cause a false reading. The healthcare team is attuned to this possibility and will troubleshoot if the number doesn't correlate with the way your child looks. As the saturation of oxygen changes, the tone of the pulse oximeter also will change. The doctors and nurses taking care of your son or daughter are focused on these particular changes.

With all those tubes, how will my child be able to urinate?

Dr. Zucker: After open-heart surgery a child usually has a catheter (called a Foley catheter) placed through the urethra into the bladder to remove any urine. Yet another tube! The nurses and doctors monitor the amount of urine that accumulates. Often you will see many people focused on the amount of urine produced, as it helps us determine the overall functioning of the heart. A happy kidney is a happy heart, which is therefore a happy baby.

Will my child be in pain after surgery? How much pain medication will be administered?

Dr. Zucker: Heart surgery is associated with some discomfort. However, the healthcare team is quite attuned to this issue, as pain has been shown to contribute to a delayed recovery. So after heart surgery children either receive pain medications through the IV, as needed, or on a continuous basis. The team can determine pain and discomfort even when the child is unable to tell us. Heart rate and blood pressure are factors in this assessment. We also look at the size of the pupils, which, in part, is the reason why nurses shine a light into your child's eyes. If you feel that your child is in pain based on appearance or "inside information" about how your child responds to discomfort, please let your nurse or doctor know.

Many intravenous pain-relief medications, particularly narcotics, are apt to slow the respiratory rate. We try to balance pain management with our efforts to remove the child from the ventilator.

What is a ventilator? Why does my child need one after surgery?

Dr. Zucker: A ventilator goes by several names, including "respirator" and "breathing machine." After heart surgery, the team may determine that the child's recovery would be better served by several hours to several days of respiratory support through the use of a ventilator. Since breathing takes a fair amount of energy and pain medications can slow the breathing rate, we often utilize the ventilator to deliver the oxygen and remove the carbon dioxide. There are many types of ventilators, many different modes, and most notably many different alarms. You will notice that the doctor and respiratory therapist will spend a fair amount of time adjusting the ventilator to optimize your child's lung function.

How do you know that a child is ready to come off the ventilator? How do you get my child off the ventilator?

Dr. Zucker: After your child wakes up from surgery, she will start to breathe more on her own. The team will slowly decrease the number of breaths the machine gives as your child does more of the lungs' work on her own. We measure the effectiveness of the child's efforts by taking blood from the arterial line to look at the amount of oxygen and carbon dioxide in the blood. When these numbers are ideal and when no other contraindications exist, we remove the breathing tube (also known as extubation). Some doctors prefer to have the child breathe through the endotracheal tube without the assistance of any breaths from the machine prior to extubation. This is known as CPAP (continuous positive airway pressure). Others choose to remove the breathing tube after the machine has been decreased to a few breaths per minute.

"Before they removed Lissie's breathing tube, they wanted her to be fully awake. Unfortunately, she was very uncomfortable and crying inconsolably. Mat and I tried every form of distraction—singing her favorite songs, reading her favorite books. . . . Finally, Carolyn, her nurse, suggested we step away and let her give it a try. When we got back, the tube had been removed and Lissie was lying there happily."

—Shari Maurer, mom to Lissie (tetralogy of Fallot)

"He stopped breathing about two weeks after his surgery, after he was taken off a ventilator and while he was still in the hospital. He was resuscitated and taken back to intensive care. It was awful for us because I had been feeling pretty good about his being ready to come home and now I was convinced this would happen at home."

—Anne Linne, mom to Kevin (transposition of the great vessels)

"After Seth's first surgery they had removed his chest tube and his lung collapsed and the tube had to be reinserted. The nurses were wonderful but they did say, 'Don't worry, this happens all the time.' Well, I was worried and it didn't happen all the time to me."

—Shelly Corush, mom to Seth (coarctation of the aortic artery, ASDs, VSDs, surgical heart block with a pacemaker)

What is an arterial line?

Dr. Zucker: An arterial line is a catheter (a piece of plastic) that is placed into the artery to measure blood pressure and obtain blood for tests.

Similar to the IV catheters that are in the veins, this catheter is often in the radial artery or sometimes in the femoral artery (in the groin). You may see blood in the tube of the arterial line, as sampling of blood is necessary to determine the child's oxygen level, carbon dioxide level, hematocrit (which determines whether the baby is anemic), and chemistry levels. Samples from the arterial line often limit the need to obtain blood from veins and also decrease the chance that your child will need to be "stuck" for blood. We usually remove arterial lines shortly after the child goes off the ventilator. Although the line essentially eliminates the need to draw blood from the veins, for safety reasons arterial lines are not used in the regular inpatient areas of the hospital and must be removed before leaving the intensive care unit or step-down area.

What is a blood gas?

Dr. Zucker: Blood gases are obtained from either an artery or a vein. Essentially they have three components: pH, PaO_2, and PCO_2. The pH measures the amount of acid or base in the bloodstream. Much like pH sampling performed to maintain swimming pools, optimum performance of the human body requires maintaining the pH in a narrow range. Low pH's reflect increased acid buildup, and high pH's reflect increased base buildup. Acid buildup can be from an ineffective removal of carbon dioxide from the lungs or due to acid production from the tissues of the body. To correct these problems we can adjust the ventilator or administer bicarbonate to buffer the acid.

PCO_2 is the partial pressure of carbon dioxide in the blood. It is the measure of the effectiveness of the ventilation in concert with the child's effort to remove the CO_2 produced by his or her body.

The PaO_2 is the partial pressure of oxygen and may range from the 30s to the 400 to 500s, depending on many factors. Newborns with complex heart disease may have PaO_2s in the low range due to the anatomy of the heart, whereas others may have very high PaO_2s when supplemental oxygen is administered.

In an effort to avoid frequent blood sampling from the arterial line, we measure oxygen saturation with a pulse oximeter to determine the oxygen level in the blood. It does not, however, tell us the pH or the PCO_2. We don't focus on a specific number; we assess many variables to determine whether the blood gases are at the levels they should be.

What is an oxygen tent used for?

Dr. Zucker: After removing the tracheal tube, we may place the child in a tent for supplemental oxygen. Many infants and children don't cooperate with us when we try to put an oxygen mask on their face, so we use oxygen tents instead. In addition, they can act as humidifiers, which may help reduce discomfort from irritation of the trachea during intubation. As with every other aspect of postoperative care, the oxygen tent would be tailored to your individual child's needs.

Why do they keep X-raying my child?

Dr. Zucker: X rays help the team evaluate many different problems. X rays will reveal whether there is any fluid in or around the lungs or the heart, any signs of lung infection, positioning of the tracheal tube and important catheters and drains, as well as changes in the size of the heart. Comparison with a previous day's films is helpful when evaluating potential changes. X rays sometimes lag behind the clinical picture by a day or so, but they are very helpful to your child's doctor and nurse.

Why are they banging on my child's back?

Dr. Zucker: Many doctors believe that chest physiotherapy (banging on your child's back with either a cupped hand or an anesthesia mask) helps mobilize the secretions that are in your child's lungs. Interestingly, many children find this soothing rather than uncomfortable. After chest PT, your child may cough and clear the mucus that has accumulated in his windpipe and lungs during surgery. As your child improves, the frequency of chest PT is decreased.

Why do some children run fevers after surgery? Is this dangerous? What does it mean? Can I take my child home if he has a fever?

Dr. Zucker: It's a misconception that all fevers are related to infection. In actual fact, fever is the body's ability to respond to any stress, whether it be from infection or just increased metabolism due to various components of recovery. The most common reason for children to have fever after surgery is as the result of collapse of some of the air sacs of the lung. By and large this is not a major concern and often resolves within a day or two after surgery. Usually, with deep breaths, sitting up in bed, and chest physiotherapy, these small air sacs pop back open and the fever disappears. The doctors and nurses watch a fever closely because of the more dire possibilities of infection and/or fluid sitting around the heart or around the lungs. Various tests (including X rays, echocardiograms, and blood tests) are key to differentiating between or among the different causes of fever after heart surgery. Efforts should be made by all of the healthcare team to help delineate the cause of the increased temperature, as it may contribute to a delay in recovery and discharge. Usually a feverish child would not be discharged, however, on a rare occasion if the cause is identified and the healthcare team is comfortable with postoperative follow-up, she may be sent home.

How can I ensure that my milk supply still comes in when I won't be able to breast-feed right away?

Dr. Zucker: The effects of the anesthesia often will depress a child's normal bowel activity. Therefore, food—whether it be breast milk or table food—may not be adequately digested, so during the first twelve to twenty-four hours after heart surgery, we are often hesitant to feed children. Some exceptions to this are operations that allow for early extubation (removal of the tracheal tube) so feedings can occur sooner. Medications often contribute to the decreased bowel activity. By the first to second day after the operation, babies and children can usually begin to take food by mouth or through a nasogastric (NG) or nasoduodenal (ND) tube (a small plastic tube placed through the nose into the stomach or duodenum). At that time, breast milk can be administered through either the NG or ND tube or directly from the breast. To assure that Mom's milk supply is still available when her baby is ready for it, we recommend that she pump her breasts and store the milk for later use.

"When Zachary was at the other hospital having his surgery, I thought that I wouldn't breast-feed him. I asked the nurse for ice packs to help dry up the milk. She wouldn't give them to me, instead encouraging me to pump so I would be able to nurse him when he was ready. I pumped until he was ten days old. I will never forget when they handed him to me and I breast-fed him for the first time. He was ten days old and I realized I had never even held him before."

—Carole Stoll, mom to Zachary
(VSD, subaortic stenosis, interrupted aortic arch)

When can I hold my child?

Dr. Zucker: The physical bond between parents and their children is most beneficial in the healing process. If doctors and nurses hesitate to allow parents to hold their child, it's for purely practical reasons. Once many of the catheters and the tracheal tubes are removed, the potential for dislodgment of an important IV is obviously decreased and we encourage parents to cuddle and touch their child. At times it may be necessary to keep certain catheters or tubes in place, but cautiously placing the child in the parent's arms remains a possibility. Since the routine postoperative patient doesn't require prolonged cardiac or respiratory support, it usually takes but a few days before the child is up and about and his parents can hold him freely.

"As soon as you can, participate in the normal hygiene routine of your child. Take part in bathing, diaper changes, dressing, etc. After a while, especially for parents of a newborn, it can feel like your baby belongs to the nurses. Don't forget that you are Mommy and Daddy and your child needs you. Your role is very important in healing and recovery."

—*Susie DeLoach, mom to Joey (HLHS)*

The Recovery Floor

How do the doctors decide when my child is ready to leave the ICU?

Dr. Zucker: The decision to leave the ICU is based on several factors. First, a child remains in the ICU until the vital signs (heart rate, blood pressure, respiratory rate, temperature, and oxygen saturation) are normal for someone with the type of surgical repair she had. In addition, we look to be sure that there are no other problems involving the heart, lungs, kidneys, or brain. Last, we assess to be sure that pain will be optimally managed in the regular inpatient areas.

THE RECOVERY FLOOR

"Once Alex got to the floor I turned into her nurse, doctor, advocate, everything. Her roommate had a breathing problem and kept having episodes during the night that kept waking up my baby. I finally took her to the nurse's station and said 'Please find another place for us to sleep.' I felt like the mama lion fighting for her cub. But they put us in the playroom and we were able to sleep."

—*Pat Posada Klapper, mom to Alexandra (VSD)*

"Once we were moved to the recovery floor, we were allowed to sleep in the room with Max. That was a great relief!"

—*Jeff Kramer, dad to Max (tetralogy of Fallot)*

"We were really looking forward to Henry's being moved to the regular cardiac unit, but ironically, once he was moved, we were scared because he didn't receive the same twenty-four-hours-a-day-with-his-own-nurse care."

—*Laurie Strongin, mom to Henry (tetralogy of Fallot)*

"We were not prepared when our son was moved from intensive care into pediatrics. We didn't realize that one of us should stay with him because he wouldn't have a full-time nurse anymore. I felt we had to be more on top of things once he got to pediatrics."

—*Anne Linne, mom to Kevin (transposition of the great vessels)*

The nurses have asked me not to throw out my baby's diapers after changing them. Why is this? What are they looking for?

Dr. Zucker: After a child's Foley catheter is removed from the ureter, it is still important to determine how well the baby's kidneys are working. We weigh the diapers in an effort to determine how much the baby has urinated between diaper changes.

My child is a very picky eater. Will there be different types of food to choose from? Can I bring food from home for him?

Dr. Zucker: Hospital food is notorious for being less than palatable. It can turn a hearty eater picky and make an already fussy eater fussier. On top of that, the combination of medications, fatigue from surgery, and mild anemia can further diminish appetite. We encourage parents to supplement their child's hospital diet with home-cooked meals, but it's a good idea to consult your physician and the hospital nutritionist first. This would help avoid any potential contraindications to other diets, such as diets laced with extra salt and diets with heavy fat content. Unfortunately, as many hospitals have moved toward fast-food franchises in their lobbies, it's difficult to restrict what enters the mouths of many babies.

"It is sometimes very hard to control them while they're in bed, when they want to leave."

—*Sharon Popp, mom to Ben*
(pulmonary atresia with VSD, transposition of the aorta)

When can my child go to the playroom?

Dr. Zucker: Therapeutic play has been shown to decrease stress in the pre- and postoperative patient, and play is a critical component to a child's recovery. All team members are encouraged to foster this element of recuperation. It's hard for a child to leave the intensive care unit, but Child Life specialists are available to work with children at the bedside. Sometimes, after a major operation, children regress developmentally, and this may be apparent during play. Although this is usually temporary, it is worth mentioning to your healthcare team.

How can the social worker help me while my child is in the hospital?

Mr. Sklenar: Having a child with congenital heart disease will be a demanding and painful experience at times. Parents find that they have to make many changes in their daily lives to afford the time and energy needed to care for their child and family. Relationships—as important as they are in coping—inevitably feel the strain. New feelings surface but may be difficult to share. People intimately involved may feel guilty, worn out, sad, angry, excited, etc., without being able to identify why. These are normal reactions to a stressful situation and a way of beginning to cope with the demands placed on the family.

A hospital social worker is specially trained to help individuals and families learn to deal with lifestyle changes, problems, or crises (while in the hospital and also after discharge).

In the hospital, the social worker might be consulted about:

- Patient/family difficulties in adjusting to illness
- The stress of an illness
- Needs for assistance at home
- Social issues related to school
- Practical or financial needs
- Future education and vocational planning
- Other individual or family problems
- Age-appropriate counseling for children or their siblings to help them cope with the changes brought about by the diagnosis and treatment
- Helping parents cope with the stress of caring for an ill child, on top of juggling other home- and work-related responsibilities
- Providing any family member or the whole family with counseling to help foster coping and adjustment through the course of the child's illness and treatment

A referral can be made by your physician, nurse, or other healthcare professional, or you may wish to call or visit the social work department office in the hospital.

What factors go into deciding that my child is ready to leave the hospital?

Dr. Manning, Nurse Adler, and Nurse Wispé: The most important factor in determining when a child is ready to leave the hospital following cardiac surgery is that their cardiac and pulmonary statuses are satisfactory on a stable regimen of medicines. Being able to participate in age-appropriate activities is a good index of their cardiac and pulmonary state. Engaging in playroom activities and comfortable walking are appropriate for toddlers and older children. Taking in an adequate oral diet to maintain good nutrition is essential before discharge. Feeding comfortably without sweating or shortness of breath is a good index of activity tolerance in infants. Newborns should demonstrate a steady weight gain by discharge. Parents must be comfortable with what they will need to deliver at home, such as special wound care, medications, or dietary needs.

Who will give me instructions when I leave?

Dr. Manning, Nurse Adler, and Nurse Wispé: This may be different at different hospitals. One of your physicians will typically review some instructions prior to discharge. At most centers an advanced practice nurse working on the cardiology or cardiac surgery team and/or one of the staff nurses on the hospital unit will review instructions in detail with families and make sure the parents know whom to contact for questions or problems, as well as setting a schedule of follow-up appointments. In some cases specialists from nutrition services, physical or occupational therapy, home nursing care, or respiratory therapy also may give you instructions near the time of discharge.

"When you leave the hospital after the operation, walk away with a list of things that need to be done: medicines to be given, when your next doctor's appointment is, antibiotics you need to give before dentist appointments, etc. Type it up if you can and keep it with you."

—*Pat Posada Klapper, mom to Alexandra (VSD)*

CHAPTER 7
LIFE AFTER SURGERY

Betsy Adler, M.S.N., R.N., C.P.N.P.   James C. Huhta, M.D.

Woodrow Benson, M.D., Ph.D.   Michael J. Landzberg, M.D.

Jonas I. Bromberg, Psy.D.   Ranae Larsen, M.D.

Michael D. Freed, M.D.   Peter B. Manning, M.D.

Lisa Wispé, M.S.N., R.N., C.P.N.P.

As I write the beginning of this chapter, we are a few weeks away from Lissie's annual checkup. During the rest of the year it's often easy to pretend that nothing is wrong, until she gets an infection or a fever. I tend to worry a little more and get her to the doctor a little sooner than with my son, because in the back of my mind I'm not really sure when her repaired heart defect is going to influence a basic childhood illness. My pediatricians are great—they always address my concerns, and if they're not sure how something (an illness, a medication, a vaccine, etc.) will affect Lissie, they just pick up the phone and call her cardiologist.

So while the rest of our year is fairly uneventful, suddenly it's time for her checkup again, and suddenly I'm worried. What if all is not well this time? Robin Yankow, whose son Eddie has aortic stenosis and an enlarged aortic root, summed it up when she said, "About three weeks before his appointment I get wiggy and even when everything is fine, for about a week after I can't relax." The future may hand you some unexpected turns. Many children will need additional surgery or live with the knowledge that somewhere down the road they will need a transplant. Gerri's son Max was readmitted to the hospital shortly after his repair because they suspected an arrhythmia at one of his checkups (he was fine), and once for croup, which was entirely unrelated to his heart, but the fact of his repaired tetralogy unnerved the emergency room staff that was treating him.

Leaving the hospital after your child's surgery also can be a very stressful time. We heard from a lot of parents who were quite nervous about "doing it on their own" after the relative comfort of knowing that at the hospital there was always someone to back you up if you needed help. We tried to answer some basic questions about this postsurgery time, but you should know if you have any questions we didn't cover, help is probably just a phone call away—to the nurses at the hospital, your cardiologist, or your pediatrician. Never be afraid to call with a question. There are no stupid questions, and one phone call can often put your fears at ease. Lissie ran a fever a day or two after her discharge. We called our cardiologist, who suggested we bring her back to the hospital for a quick checkup, just in case. They did an exam and a few tests to rule out infection or fluid around her heart and then determined that the fever had nothing to do with her heart. But it just as easily could have been a surgical complication, so we're glad that we got her examined.

And then there's her scar, at this point a barely visible exclamation point that reminds us of her journey, though most of the time we don't even notice it. At five years old, it's not a big concern to her—just a normal part of her body. I don't know how she will feel when she gets older, but almost every one of the parents we heard from said that their child felt their scar was no big deal.

Even when all seems well, we still worry. And that's okay. In fact, if you talk to any parent, even those whose children's hearts are fine, you know that worry is just part of everyday parenthood.

Meanwhile, in a few weeks, along with Lissie's checkup, we're going to have a fetal echo done on the baby we're expecting next spring. We'll do both exams on the same day so Lissie might feel more comfortable if she has an echo and then Mommy has an echo on the new baby, too. Although our chances are only slightly higher than the general population of having a second child with CHD, we want to reassure ourselves that this baby's heart is okay (we had a fetal echo when I was pregnant with my second child, too). And if the worst happens and this child also has a defect, we feel that, having been down the road once before, we'll figure it out.

Shari

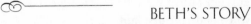

BETH'S STORY
By Beth Grampovnik, age thirteen

I have had three open-heart surgeries. I had two in Chicago, Illinois, one when I was two years old and the other when I was five years old. When I was five I had a pacemaker put in, also. I had my third surgery in New York when I was eight years old.

During my time in the hospital many things happened. When I met different doctors before my surgery I was scared and confused. But after my surgery I didn't feel afraid. I knew they had helped me.

A lot of things helped me during my time in the hospital. What helped the most were family and friends. My family would read me stories and talk to me, and I knew that they would always be there. My friends would call me. I loved when they did that. My class also sent me homemade cards that I liked a lot. Another thing that helped was talking to the doctors and asking them questions, so I knew what was going on. The surgeries affected me a lot. I went through something tough and I made it. I know I have more courage and bravery than before my surgery. I can do things better, too. I got much stronger. I am in seventh grade and I have played basketball and volleyball for two years on my school team. I got MIP (Most Improved Player) awards once in volleyball and once in basketball. I swim and run around with my friends. I can do the same things my friends do even though I have had three heart surgeries. I feel I can do anything, after what I have been through. Anybody can do anything!

Activity

What are the most common restrictions given to children after heart surgery?

Dr. Manning, Nurse Adler, and Nurse Wispé: All children should follow some restrictions for a period of four to six weeks following surgery simply to ensure good wound healing. Specific recommendations will vary depending on the child's age. Activities that invite the possibility of a blow to the incision area should be avoided. This includes roughhousing with friends, siblings, or pets; and climbing or playing on toys that could possibly result in a fall. Lifting or carrying heavy objects also should be avoided. This includes heavy books or backpacks for school-age children. A child should *not* remain inactive during the recovery period. Aerobic activities such as walking or swimming are excellent for heart and lung recovery after surgery. Climbing stairs is fine as long as a child is not too winded by the exercise. Range-of-motion or stretching activities are helpful to avoid stiffness.

"Brian just got a skateboard for his fourth birthday. He rides his bike and can hit a baseball over the house and hang from the monkey bars. When the doctor saw him the other day he said, 'There's my superman. All he needs is his cape.'"

—*Laura Ulaszek, mom to Brian (HLHS)*

Is it safe for my postop child to climb and stretch? What are the dangers if she falls?

Dr. Manning, Nurse Adler, and Nurse Wispé: Stretching and flexibility exercises are good after surgery. Climbing can be a problem if a child loses her balance and falls. Falling can obviously be painful soon after an operation. A severe fall could strain an incision enough to result in weakening the incision or slowing the healing process.

My doctor told me my daughter shouldn't overexert herself. Does that apply only to activities such as running and jumping? What about if she gets angry and throws a tantrum? Is she overexerting herself then?

Dr. Manning, Nurse Adler, and Nurse Wispé: Throwing a tantrum may be more exertion than we would normally like to see in the early postoperative period, but if a child has enough energy to get that worked up, it's usually a good sign that his or her cardiac energy reserve is returning to normal. It is important for parents to stick to the same rules of behavior after surgery as before. Spoiling a child excessively or bending the rules around the time of surgery can result in many more problems, including tantrums, when you try to return to the "old rules."

How soon after surgery can most kids take a tub bath or go swimming?

Dr. Manning, Nurse Adler, and Nurse Wispé: In some cases a tub bath or swimming is okay a week after surgery. The concern about tub baths or swimming is the possibility of heavy and prolonged exposure of the incision to germs that may increase the risk of infection. Because some monitors or drains aren't removed until a few days after an operation, it's usually safest to wait until the Steri-Strips are off before long tub baths or swimming.

How soon after surgery can most kids resume normal activity?

Dr. Manning, Nurse Adler, and Nurse Wispé: Normal activities such as going to school or day care may often resume a week or two after discharge. Activities that could result in a fall or a blow to the area of the incision, or heavy lifting should be avoided for four to six weeks following surgery. After this time, return to any activity is generally okay, unless the child has been restricted by his doctor for some reason.

How soon after coming home from the hospital can my child play with her friends?

Dr. Freed: After coming home from the hospital, many children want to get back to their normal life as soon as possible. Since so much of children's play involves others, there is a natural tendency to want to have company. For most children, this interaction speeds the recuperation. As long as others do not have signs of active infection (runny nose, cough, fever, vomiting, diarrhea, etc.), we usually allow the children to play with their siblings immediately and with friends and relatives within a few days of going home.

"For nearly three months after surgery, Alex was very clingy. He only wanted Mom (occasionally Dad was okay, too). He wanted to be held constantly, and he would cry when he was with other people. As a stay-at-home mom, I was able to be with Alex and take the time to hold him and reassure him. After about three months he started feeling more secure again and also felt a lot better physically and so became much more active and outgrew his clingy stage."

—Sara Daniel, mom to Alex (tricuspid atresia, ASD, VSD)

"The day Lissie came home from the hospital, she was running through the hallways of our apartment building, like nothing had happened."

—Shari Maurer, mom to Lissie (tetralogy of Fallot)

"Isaiah's second surgery (Glenn shunt) was completed at seven months of age. . . . While his physical recovery was excellent—just five days—his emotional recovery was still ongoing even after one month postop. In fact, one day after we were released from the hospital, Isaiah stopped drinking from the bottle and would refuse his meds from a syringe. We had to take him back to UCLA the next morning because he was getting dehydrated. We were able to determine (though the doctors still are not convinced of this) that Isaiah finally had enough of people sticking things in his mouth. . . . We began mixing his meds with his baby food and we backed off on the 'force feedings' and offered him a bottle only when he was hungry. The next day he was fine and we were on our way home."

—Randy Sittner, dad to Isaiah
(hypoplastic right ventricle, pulmonary atresia, and tricuspid atresia)

When can my child go back to school?

Dr. Freed: Depending upon the speed of recuperation, some children want to go back almost immediately. We usually recommend at least the first week at home. Some children are ready to go back to school the second week. If there is any question, it is sometimes helpful to start school part-time for the first week, either by starting with a half day or a full day every other day.

My child's condition was surgically repaired. Do I need to inform the school? We've been told that he has no physical restrictions, so I really don't think it's necessary.

Dr. Larsen: Even if your child has no known residual heart problems and does not require restrictions of his activity level, the school should be informed of his cardiac history. The risk of late or long-term problems is low with many types of repaired heart defects, but some problems such as rhythm disturbances may occur. The school should be informed that your child should be allowed to rest during or after physical activities if he becomes excessively tired, or if he develops dizziness, palpitations, or chest pain. If your child became ill at school and required treatment, the history of congenital heart disease might be very important in the child's evaluation and treatment by school and medical personnel.

If your child receives any medications, even if none of them is given at school, the school should be aware of the medications, their doses, the times when they are given, and the reason or reasons the medications are given. If you are told of potential side effects of the medications, these possible side effects should be relayed to the school.

Your school may find it helpful for your cardiologist to write a letter to the school nurse or to the child's teacher describing the nature of your child's heart disease; symptoms to watch for; and precautions, if any, to take.

"Our life is pretty normal now. We both work, and Shelby goes to day care every day."

—*Dan and Candy Miller, parents of Shelby (severe pulmonary stenosis)*

"Brian's preschool has been wonderful. We filled out an extensive medical history and then they asked me more questions, including his average heart rate, information on the medication he was taking, all of the phone numbers they would need—pediatrician, cardiologist, etc. We gave them copies of all of Brian's surgical reports. I keep his records updated quarterly. He's in a regular classroom doing regular stuff."

—Laura Ulaszek, mom to Brian (HLHS)

"Eddie is starting kindergarten this fall. We have met with the guidance counselor, gym teacher, nurse, and principal to give them his medical information. We have decided not to let everyone in the whole school know about Eddie's heart—we don't want him to be labeled, but we did want the key people to know so that if he complained of chest pains they should take him seriously. His teacher and I will maintain good communication so that if she sees anything concerning (like if he tires easily), she will be able to tell me. A lot of good things came out of that meeting. We got to share all of the medical stuff, but they also got a chance to get to know Eddie, too."

—Robin Yankow, mom to Eddie (aortic stenosis, enlarged aortic root)

Will my child's travel be restricted in any way?

Dr. Manning, Nurse Adler, and Nurse Wispé: Traveling can be tiring following an operation, and may take you to places where you are unfamiliar with the medical resources available and they are unfamiliar with your case. Avoid unnecessary travel until you have been back for a follow-up visit with your doctor.

Dr. Freed: For most children, recuperation after surgery is complete within two or three weeks. There are a few complications that can occur after going home. Infections may occur within the first week or two but are quite uncommon. Rarely, fluid can build up around the heart or the lungs. This complication occurs within a couple of weeks. Therefore we usually postpone vacations for about a month after surgery. When you go away, you should know how to contact your pediatric cardiologist and may want to get the name of a pediatric cardiologist in the area where the vacation is planned.

My child had open-heart surgery as a baby. Can she play contact sports (football, hockey, etc.)?

Dr. Larsen: A child's participation in contact sports depends upon the age of the child, the type of congenital heart disease, whether there are any significant residual heart defects, the types of medications your child may be taking, and the specific type of sports considered. You should discuss with your child's doctor whether your child is at increased risk from physical contact. Many children with repaired congenital heart disease don't have restrictions on their participation in sports. Exercise and sports recommendations should be tailored to each individual child, however. Your pediatric cardiologist should be able to tell you exactly what types of activities are safe for your child. An exercise test or echocardiogram may be needed to assist your doctor in determining the types and level of activities that are appropriate for your child.

Contact sports should be avoided with some kinds of defects and problems. Patients with pacemakers should avoid contact sports, because trauma may break the pacemaker leads and cause the pacemaker to malfunction. Patients with artificial valves are often on anticoagulation medications such as warfarin (Coumadin) to prevent the valve from developing blood clots around it. These patients bleed more easily than normal, and trauma may cause life-threatening bleeding. Patients with Marfan syndrome have an abnormality of their blood vessel walls, which makes them prone to dilatation and rupture of their aorta. Patients with Marfan must not participate in activities in which there is likely to be traumatic physical contact.

Some children also require restrictions in their participation in noncontact sports. Your cardiologist will be able to evaluate your child and recommend exercises and physical activities specific for your child.

How can competitive sports affect a young adult with CHD?

Dr. Landzberg: The ultimate test of the efficiency of the cardiopulmonary system and its interaction with the body is athletics.

Your approach toward competitive athletics mandates a continued relationship with and guidance from a CHD specialist. While the American Heart Association and the American College of Cardiology have clear and specific recommendations for allowances and limitations of athletics for various degrees of medical illness associated with CHD, these are at best guidelines to be read and serve as an introduction. Individual diagnoses and medical histories may mandate only further instruction and training in some circumstances, while others may require special testing.

At present, many young adults with CHD have had interventions designed to further maximize their cardiopulmonary capacity. While greatest risk appears centered in those persons with hypertrophic cardiomyopathy, congenital "long QT syndrome," congenital coronary artery anomalies, Marfan disease, myocarditis, pulmonary hypertension, right ventricular dysplasia, and Kawasaki disease with associated aneurysm formation, particular limitations to exercise capacity continue to exist for other adults with CHD. Effects of excessive heart muscle development (ventricular hypertrophy) and enlargement (dilatation), abnormal or even bypassed (Fontan) right ventricular function, and relatively immobile pulmonary artery resistance in some persons with pulmonary hypertension, and cyanosis, combine to further limit persons with CHD.

GETTING PHYSICAL

"Scott has always been encouraged to set his own levels and to rest when he felt he needed it. His teachers and day-care providers have always been told not to 'push' him, but not to 'baby' him either. So far it's worked well. Empowering the child is very beneficial."

—Sue Dove, mom to Scott (single ventricle)

"We steered Johnny into nonphysical things like bowling, golf, things he will always be able to do. He's very involved in Scouts and school activities other than athletics. Johnny became an Eagle Scout on March 25, 1998, three weeks before open-heart surgery. What an accomplishment!!!"

—Sandra Gravel, mom to Johnny
(coarctation, aortic stenosis, subaortic stenosis)

"[You can help your child] by letting them be themselves and knowing their own limitations and not placing limitations on them, which is very hard for parents to do because it is a natural thing . . . to be overprotective."

—Brian Susnis, dad to Taylor (VSD, interrupted aortic arch)

"At this time she is not allowed to run the mile at school. She is only to walk. The gym teacher allows another child to walk with her, which helps."

—Sheryl Lamb, mom to Heather (double outlet right ventricle,
hypoplastic right upper chamber, transposition,
subvalvular pulmonary stenosis, bilateral superior vena cava with
interrupted inferior vena cava, common ventricle)

"Physical limitations are noticeable if he's running around with kids and he stops more to rest. He also doesn't walk as far as our other child."

—Sharon Popp, mom to Ben
(pulmonary atresia with VSD, transposition of the aorta)

"Allowing adequate rest and a quiet home seems especially important to Alyssa, which is different from other kids her age."

—Sylvia Paul, mom to Alyssa (tricuspid atresia)

"Because he's not allowed to participate in contact sports, we've gotten Eddie involved in a swim program. He's taken off like a natural. We are so thrilled."

—Robin Yankow, mom to Eddie (aortic stenosis and enlarged aortic root)

Are there any special camps for children with CHD? What are the benefits of these camps?

Dr. Landzberg: Depending upon the time of year, newspapers and the Internet are filled with advertisements for summer camps that either incorporate or are "designed" for children and adolescents with "special needs." Summer fun and accomplishments with similarly aged children allow for growth, independence, self-worth, and sense of community, and are benefits in whatever venue they are offered. The experiences of campers are nearly universally felt to be excellent, though long-term results are unknown, as the camps are relatively new in existence. Scholarships are frequently available. (See Resources for a list of some camps for CHD kids.)

"The very best thing about camp was that I got to be with other kids who are just like me. They made me feel really good because it's like we're all in the same world and we all know just how each other feels. It's a lot harder to be with kids who aren't like me because they make me feel really different. They say 'What are those?' about the scars on my chest, and what I always say is 'See ya tomorrow, I'll tell ya then!' I get so tired of kids staring and asking me questions. But at camp I could just be me; I didn't even cover up my scars when I went swimming! No one made fun of anyone else. No one stared. That's because at camp, every kid has something wrong with him. Every single one of us."

—Gavin Dehler, eleven years old
(Orlando, Florida, Boggy Creek Hole In the Wall Gang camper)

"It's kind of a club here. It's their special place that no one else can come to."
—Jerri Clifford, R.N. (nurse at the Edward Madden Open Hearts Camp)

"I met my best friend at this camp—I've known her for eight years. It's nice here because I'm never embarrassed by being tired. You can rest."

—Nora Shimmel, sixteen years old
(transposition of the great vessels, pacemaker;
Edward Madden Open Hearts Camp camper and staff member)

Scars

How do I care for my son's incision? Can it get wet? Will the Steri-Strip fall off, or do I need to remove it? Is there danger if the incision is exposed to the sun? Is there anything I can do to minimize scarring?

Dr. Manning, Nurse Adler, and Nurse Wispé: The most important aspect of caring for an incision after surgery is to keep it clean. Washing at least once a day with soap and water is usually allowed at the time of discharge from the hospital. Most physicians will recommend that you don't soak the area of the incision (such as in a bathtub or swimming pool) for at least a week after surgery, but sponge bathing or showering is generally fine by the time of hospital discharge. Steri-Strips will usually start to peel off after a week or so. It's okay to remove them when they have separated from the area of the incision itself. If they are still on by the time of your first return appointment to the doctor, they will usually be removed then. Healing tissue such as surgical incisions are more sensitive to sun damage than normal skin. They should be protected from excessive exposure to the sun, and high SPF sunblock should be used as long as the scar has any pink color (this may be for a number of months in some cases). Everyone scars differently, and some factors are beyond anyone's control. Preventing infection or other damage to the healing area is the most important factor in avoiding an unsightly scar. Applying creams with vitamins or other factors is advocated by some, but there is little strong evidence that they significantly affect the scarring process. Creams containing steroids should be avoided, as these impair the wound healing and infection resistance of the skin.

Is there any way to minimize scarring or to remove a scar? I see all sorts of advertisements for creams, Vitamin E, laser surgery. Can I believe any of it?

Dr. Larsen: There is no way to completely remove a scar, but there are methods to try to minimize the prominence of the scar. Care of the wound immediately after surgery is of utmost importance. Keep the chest incision clean, dry, and open to air, unless otherwise specified by your surgeon. Your child should bathe daily in a shower or a tub with gentle soap and water to keep the incision free of infection. Many surgeons close the skin with under-the-skin absorbable sutures that do not require removal. Most of these scars heal with a thin, flat scar. If there are signs of infection, such as reddening of the surrounding skin, swelling, a new separation of the wound, or drainage, notify your surgeon immediately, as the child may be developing a wound infection. An infected wound will not heal well and may result in a prominent scar.

After any scabbing has resolved, aloe vera or vitamin E cream applied daily for two to four months may help soften the scar and aid in healing. Also, silicone sheeting applied daily during this same period may keep the scar from being raised and prominent. Silicone sheeting is available over-the-counter in many pharmacies. Both the creams and the silicone sheeting may decrease the risk of keloid formation.

Keloid scars are thickened, raised, wide, and often tender scars that occur in some children and adults. They can be difficult to treat once they occur. Silicone sheeting placed daily for several months may aid in flattening keloids. Other keloids or prominent scars may be treated by surgical excision and revision or by removal with a laser by a plastic surgeon.

My daughter has a scar from her open-heart surgery and doesn't want to get undressed in front of the other girls for gym class. What can I do to help her with this?

Dr. Larsen: Explain to your child, in a way that's appropriate to her age, the reason for the scar so that she feels comfortable with her history of heart disease and surgery. She should be able to tell her classmates briefly about the reasons for the scar. If your child has a best friend, an explanation to that friend by a parent and/or the child may give support within your child's circle of friends and acquaintances. Children are naturally curious about differences among them. Once friends and classmates have an explanation, they are usually matter-of-fact and accepting. Your child may even be proud of her scar as something special, unique, and interesting about her. It's important that parents feel comfortable with the scar; anxious or negative feelings may inadvertently be transmitted to the child. If the parents are accepting of the scar; children will often follow their lead.

COPING WITH SCARS

"Robby's scar story . . . he would tell everyone he had survived a major shark attack and the shark didn't make it. He was actually upset that they cut over his first scar. The chest tube scars were teeth marks. . . . Robby showed my Cub Scouts his scar and the boys all thought it was cool and Robby was brave."

—*Pamela Kostrzewa, mom to Robby* (severe aortic stenosis, mitral insufficiency, severe aortic regurgitation)

"We bought a Madeline doll with a scar and read the book about Madeline's appendectomy. I loved the scene where Madeline shows off her scar and all the other children are envious. I think this really affected my daughter and explains her pride when she shows it off (even at almost eight years old)."

—*Karen Dahlman, mom to Rebecca (ASD)*

"I know that when Joey is older, I'll tell him to be proud of his scar and what he's been through. I'll tell him how tough he is and how proud we are of him. I'll hopefully be able to teach him not to let insensitive comments from others get to him."

—*Susie DeLoach, mom to Joey (HLHS)*

"When Christina was little, the fact that she had a big scar down the middle of her chest bothered her—she didn't like to show it or for people to ask her about it. As she has gotten older, it doesn't seem to bother her."

—*Deanna Lopez, mom to Christina*
(pulmonary atresia stenosis, pacemaker)

"We were at the clinic, and the nurse was asking Scott what was wrong. He filled her in on his ear infection, but then when she asked if he was on any meds, I said, 'Yes, he's a heart patient.' She said 'Really! Me, too!!' and proceeded to pull up her shirt a little bit and compare scars with Scott!! She has had a valve replaced in her heart three times, she said. She told Scott that they could be 'scar twins.' I thought it was cool that she was willing to share that, and it was great for Scott to see an adult with heart-related scars."

—*Sue Dove, mom to Scott (single ventricle)*

"Max was talking to his fourteen-year-old female cousin, whom he was a little in awe of, and they were talking about the Backstreet Boys. Her favorite one was Nick. Max said his favorite one was Brian. Then he held open the collar of his shirt and said, 'See this? Brian has one, too!' "

—*Jeff Kramer, dad to Max (tetralogy of Fallot)*

Medical Concerns and Complications

What do I do if my child gets a fever after he's home from the hospital?

Dr. Manning, Nurse Adler, and Nurse Wispé: Low-grade fevers are relatively common in the first week or two following surgery and often are related to minor lung collapse from not taking deep breaths. A fever above 101°F or one that persists after a dose of Tylenol may indicate something more serious. Check the incision for any swelling or redness of the surrounding skin (this includes sites where drains or IVs were). If a child's appetite or activity level seems different with the fever, this also would raise concerns. Don't hesitate to call your primary care physician or someone on the cardiac team if you have *any* questions about infections.

What are the common complications or things I should look out for?

Dr. Manning, Nurse Adler, and Nurse Wispé: Wound infections and pericardial effusions are two of the more severe problems that may become evident after discharge. Signs of infection include fever, redness, swelling or pain at the site of the incision (don't forget to check the drain and IV sites also). Pericardial effusions (fluid accumulated around the heart) can cause fevers, shortness of breath, or loss of energy and can be easily diagnosed by echocardiography. Gastrointestinal problems, especially constipation related to the effects of narcotic pain medications, are common in children after surgery.

I live far from the hospital. If something goes wrong, is it better for me to call my local doctor or one of the doctors who cared for him at the hospital?

Dr. Manning, Nurse Adler, and Nurse Wispé: If you feel your child needs to be seen by a physician immediately, you should go to your local doctor or an emergency facility close to home. Most problems that may develop in the first weeks after an operation are directly associated with the surgery, but common childhood illnesses *can* occur. Hospitalization and surgery reduce a child's defenses against "routine" illnesses, and increase his or her exposure to the organisms that cause them. It is always reasonable and often wise to at least call someone familiar with your child's case at the hospital where the operation was performed if you experience problems in the first two or three weeks after discharge. If the problem sounds like one that your local physician could see, the hospital will recommend this. *Never* hesitate to call if you have any questions or concerns.

My doctor said my child will need medications for a few months after surgery. Why?

Dr. Freed: While surgery is done to palliate or correct congenital heart disease, it is nevertheless sometimes traumatic for the heart, so medications are sometimes needed temporarily after surgery. The heart muscle may be temporarily damaged by an incision made in the heart muscle during repair. And sometimes the repair increases the work of the heart by changing the blood flow. That can make one of the heart chambers work harder than it had before. Additionally, the heart/lung machine, for reasons that are not completely clear, tends to cause some fluid retention. For these reasons it may be helpful to assist the heart with medicines that increase the efficiency of the heart or get rid of excess fluid.

What is Propranolol, and why does my child need it after surgery? Do all children need it?

Dr. Freed: Propranolol is a member of a class of drugs called beta-blockers. They reduce the effects of circulating adrenaline (epinephrine) and may be used to control blood pressure or arrythmias. It may be helpful in the postoperative period in a small number of children.

What are anticoagulants, and what are they used for?

Dr. Freed: Anticoagulants are sometimes called "blood thinners," although they do not really thin the blood. Rather, they affect some of the clotting factors within the blood so that the blood is less likely to clot. They are used in some circumstances where blood has an increased tendency to form clots, most commonly when artificial, mechanical valves are used, when the heart circulation is somewhat slow (e.g., after the Fontan operation), or when there has been evidence of prior abnormal clotting.

Can my child play contact sports if he is on an anticoagulant?

Dr. Freed: Because of the reduced ability of the blood to clot, contact sports such as football or hockey are not recommended. Other sports such as baseball, basketball, tennis, etc., are not precluded.

Why is a child's blood pressure sometimes higher after surgery than before? Will this go away?

Dr. Freed: After repair of one type of congenital defect (coarctation of the aorta) the blood pressure sometimes is higher after surgery than before. This is due to a readjustment by the nervous system and/or kidneys to the surgery. It rarely lasts more than a few weeks. The blood pressure after other kinds of surgery may be elevated because of circulating adrenaline (epinephrine) due to the stress of the surgery or anxiety of the child.

My child has a fever. Is this cause for more worry than in a child without CHD?

Dr. Larsen: Usually after repair of a congenital heart defect, fever in a child with congenital heart disease has the same implications as in children without congenital heart disease and can be treated in a similar manner. Children with heart disease can, of course, have the same sorts of illnesses, such as ear infections, colds, or gastrointestinal illnesses, as normal children. Most of these infections should be evaluated and treated by your child's pediatrician or family physician as if your child had never had congenital heart disease. There are several important exceptions.

Early after surgery: Fever must be taken seriously during the first four to six weeks after surgery. During this time a child who has had open-heart surgery may develop an infection related to his surgery. If a child develops fever after heart surgery, parents should notify the child's surgeon or cardiologist so it can be determined whether the fever might be related to the heart surgery. Two causes of fever after surgery are wound infections or postpericardiotomy syndrome.

After heart surgery, a child may develop a wound infection at the site of the incision. With a wound infection, the wound may be red, swollen, excessively tender, or have a discharge of pus. Wound infections often require treatment with intravenous antibiotics, but in mild cases may need only a course of oral antibiotics. Wound infections usually occur a week to a month after surgery.

Children also may develop a complication of surgery called postpericardiotomy syndrome (PPS) after surgery. With PPS the child develops fever and often fatigue, chest pain, irritability, and poor appetite. It may occur in as many as a quarter of children older than two years of age after open-heart surgery. It is rare in children younger than two years. PPS usually occurs one to six weeks after surgery. An echocardiogram often shows fluid around the child's heart. The cause of PPS is unknown, but is felt to be due to inflammation of the pericardium or fibrous sac around the heart. PPS usually disappears on its own, but your doctor may prescribe an anti-inflammatory medicine such as aspirin, ibuprofen, or prednisone. Occasionally enough fluid accumulates around the heart that drainage through a needle or a catheter is required.

Immune deficiency: Children with deficiency of their immune system must be watched more closely than children whose immune systems are normal. Most children with congenital heart disease have normal immune systems. If your child has had a heart transplant, however, he or she is taking medicines that decrease the immune response and is more prone to serious infections than normal children. Other uncommon immune problems in children with congenital heart disease include those with asplenia or DiGeorge syndrome. Children with asplenia are born without spleens, and are more prone to certain types of infections than are normal children.

Children without spleens should receive an antibiotic such as amoxicillin or penicillin daily to avoid infection. Children with DiGeorge syndrome are born with deficiency of their lymphocytes and also are more prone to serious infection. Fevers in any immune deficient child must be taken very seriously and require immediate evaluation.

Prolonged fevers: Fevers that last more than five days with no known reason also are of concern in children with repaired congenital heart disease. Prolonged fevers without an apparent source such as an ear infection or upper respiratory infection may indicate infectious endocarditis. Infectious endocarditis is a serious condition in which there is an infection of the lining of the heart, cardiac valves, or within the major blood vessels around the heart.

Fever with infectious endocarditis is usually low-grade and is often associated with other symptoms such as fatigue, weight loss, or poor appetite. Children with congenital heart disease who are at no higher risk than the general population for the development of infective endocarditis include patients with a repaired patent ductus arteriosus, ventricular septal defect, or atrial septal defect with no residual defect. Most children with congenital heart disease, such as those with repaired tetralogy of Fallot or transposition of the great arteries, are at only mildly increased risk of endocarditis. Children at highest risk of endocarditis are those with an artificial heart valve or shunts. Children at risk for endocarditis require antibiotics before certain types of procedures such as dental work. It is key that children with congenital heart disease receive regular dental care. Poor dental health and hygiene are associated with the development of endocarditis.

Every time my child gets sick, my pediatrician acts overly cautious. Is this necessary?

Dr. Larsen: Many children with repaired congenital heart disease with no or only minimal residual cardiac disease can be treated similarly to children with no history of heart disease. Children with immune system problems (as described above), fevers lasting more than five days (without an obvious cause), or residual heart problems do need more careful evaluation and treatment than normal children. Children who receive digoxin or diuretics (water pills such as Lasix [furosemide]) may be prone to dehydration or abnormalities of their electrolytes (e.g., potassium or sodium) during episodes of vomiting, diarrhea, or decreased oral intake. Children receiving these medications may need to have the medication discontinued or decreased.

In what ways might a common virus or bacterial infection become a serious problem for a child with CHD? What common viruses and bacterial infections need to be watched with special care? What should we be watching for?

Dr. Larsen: Most infections in most children with repaired congenital heart disease can be treated in an identical manner as in healthy children without congenital heart disease. Similarly, bacterial or viral infections that are serious in children without congenital heart disease are also serious in children after repaired congenital heart disease. As previously noted, children with problems with their immune systems are at special risk from many bacterial and viral infections. Children with residual heart problems (e.g., a leaky valve or problems with heart muscle contraction) may be at increased risk for some types of infection.

Respiratory illnesses are of particular concern in children with residual cardiac defects. Respiratory syncytial virus (RSV) is a common respiratory virus often occurring during winter or early spring months. It causes an infection of the lungs called bronchiolitis. Children with bronchiolitis may have prominent wheezing and rapid breathing. Cyanosis may occur even in children who are usually pink. Children with RSV infection and cardiac disease require special observation for worsening breathing problems such as wheezing, rapid breathing, retractions (sinking in of the chest, ribs, and abdomen during breathing), and cyanosis. They often require hospitalization for respiratory care. Although RSV immune globulin and palivizumab (an anti-RSV antibody preparation) are available to decrease the risk for RSV infection in some children, neither is recommended for use in children with congenital heart disease. No immunization is available for RSV infection. Most children who have undergone repair of congenital heart disease have less severe problems than children with unrepaired or residual cardiac defects.

Children with residual congenital heart disease are also at increased risk for serious infections or complications from the influenza virus. Symptoms of flu often include a high fever, cough, and respiratory symptoms as described with RSV infection. Your pediatric cardiologist may recommend that your child receive the flu vaccine each winter.

It is very important that children with congenital heart disease receive the standard childhood immunizations as recommended by the American Academy of Pediatrics. Children with immune deficiencies may require some alteration in the immunization regimen. Check with your child's primary physician and pediatric cardiologist for specific recommendations if your child is immune-deficient.

If my pediatrician is treating my child for a virus or bacterial infection, should I call my cardiologist also?

Dr. Larsen: After repair of congenital heart disease, nearly all common viral or bacterial infections can be treated by your pediatrician or family doctor without consulting your cardiologist. Exceptions may include infections that cause severe respiratory symptoms such as wheezing, fast breathing, and retractions, or infections in children with significant residual heart defects or immune deficiencies. Patients who are receiving heart medications may need to check with their cardiologist to make sure that any medication being prescribed by their doctor for the infection doesn't interfere with the heart medication. Heart medications of particular concern include digoxin and warfarin (Coumadin). These drug dosages may need to be adjusted during treatment for the infection.

Medical Follow-up Care

How often will my child need to see the doctor in the first few months after surgery?

Dr. Manning, Nurse Adler, and Nurse Wispé: It depends on the type of surgery, the complexity of the heart disease, and the age of the patient. Your surgeon may want a follow-up visit within the first two weeks or so after discharge to assess wound healing and early postoperative recovery. Your cardiologist will often see you within the first month after surgery, then periodically on a less frequent basis after that, again depending on age and on complexity of the heart disorder. Your primary care physician should see your child within a week or two of discharge for newborns. Older children can typically follow their routine schedule of visits with their primary physician.

How often after surgery do most patients need an echo and EKG?

Dr. Freed: The need for further diagnostic and therapeutic studies depends a lot on the congenital cardiac defect and on the surgery that has been performed. For some of the simplest operations, echocardiography may not be necessary after surgery. For others, yearly (or occasionally more frequent) echocardiograms may be desirable. Any suggestion of a problem may make more frequent studies desirable. Since electrocardiography is easier and faster, these studies are usually done more frequently, although the need must be individualized based on the original heart condition and the surgery performed.

Will my child need other tests, and if so, what are they and why?

Dr. Freed: Further testing in addition to electrocardiograms and echocardiograms also depend on the nature of the original condition and the surgery. Some tests that may be recommended are chest X rays to evaluate the heart size, blood vessels, or congestion in the lungs; a pulse oximetry to measure the oxygen level in the blood; blood tests to see if the hemoglobin level in the blood is too low or two high; exercise tests to determine the effects of stress on the repaired heart; and twenty-four-hour Holter monitors or thirty-day event monitors to evaluate arrhythmias.

Occasionally, when echocardiography isn't sufficient to image a portion of the heart or lungs, magnetic resonance imaging (MRI) or positron emission tomography (PET) may be used.

If my child is repaired, why do we need to see the doctor once a year?

Dr. Larsen: Although the surgical repair of congenital heart disease has become very successful, some children have residual heart defects that require regular monitoring. Other heart defects have a risk of developing late problems, such as poor function of heart muscle, abnormal functioning of valves, or rhythm problems, and your child needs to be monitored for these potentially late complications after the treatment of heart disease. Your doctor will use the visits to assess the child's heart function, watch for worsening of any known residual problems, and educate parents and child about the potential impact of her specific repaired heart defect as the child grows and matures.

"Eventually Zachary will need a new valve, but after our doctor's appointment I try to put it away and not think about it for six months."

—Carole Stoll, mom to Zachary
(VSD, subaortic stenosis, interrupted aortic arch)

What tests will my child need at his yearly visit?

Dr. Larsen: The type of tests your child requires will depend upon the type of heart disease your child has, whether there are any residual heart defects, and the individual practice of your cardiologist. A child with congenital heart disease may require an electrocardiogram to assess heart rhythm, or an echocardiogram to monitor for residual heart defects and to assess heart muscle function. An exercise test, using a treadmill or a bicycle, also may give your doctor important information about the function of your child's heart, and to assess any rhythm problems that might be induced by exercise. The exercise test will make it easier for your doctor to make appropriate exercise recommendations for your child. If your child is known to have rhythm problems or if your child's type of heart disease is known to be associated with an increased risk of rhythm problems, a twenty-four-hour Holter monitor may be needed. A Holter records your child's electrocardiogram (usually via a cassette tape recorder) for twenty-four hours. The cardiologist then analyzes the tape for rhythm problems.

What else do you look for at the yearly visit?

Dr. Larsen: The yearly visit monitors how a child is relating to life after surgery. Your cardiologist will ask questions about your child's activity level; development; and symptoms such as fatigability, dizziness, or chest pain. The cardiologist may use the yearly visit to educate you and your child about the risk factors for heart disease, such as smoking, alcohol, drugs, and cholesterol. As a child becomes older, the cardiologist may discuss issues such as sexual activity, types of birth control, or pregnancy with the child.

My doctor says he still hears a slight murmur even though the surgeon says it was a definitive repair. Why is this? Will it go away, or will it always be there?

Dr. Freed: A heart murmur is caused by turbulence of blood as it flows through the heart. This noise can be seen in up to a third of children without heart disease. After reparative heart surgery, there still may be some residual turbulence as blood goes through valves, narrowed areas, or around patches. The presence of a murmur does not necessarily suggest that there is a significant residual problem.

Should I keep a copy of my child's EKG with me?

Dr. Landzberg: In an era of readily available transfer of information via fax machines, if your child maintains an appropriate relationship with both regional and local coordinated centers of expertise in CHD and has appropriate identification, then the answer is "not necessarily." Such miniaturized "critical" medical histories can be based upon individual need, as determined by the particular person, family, and medical caregiving team.

Why does my child need antibiotics for a visit to the dentist?

Dr. Landzberg: Some natural activities as well as some medical interventions release bacteria from the surfaces of the body into the bloodstream in unusually high amounts. Normally, our own immunologic defense mechanisms destroy, or "clear" the body of such free-floating potential harm, or "pathogens," before they settle within the body and begin tissue destruction. CHD may allow abnormal flow of blood to occur either within the heart, lungs, or blood vessels. This change in flow pattern may allow free-floating bacteria to evade our natural defense mechanisms, settle, and multiply, causing potentially catastrophic consequence from endocarditis, tissue abscesses, valve destruction, or embolism. With proper use of antibiotics, the risk of infection is significantly reduced.

Are there other times when she should have preventative antibiotics?

Dr. Landzberg: Recommendations for specific medical procedures that release bacteria from skin surfaces into the bloodstream in high amounts are constantly in flux, and should be addressed on a continuous basis with either your regional or your local medical caregiving center of expertise. In general, surgical procedures that require invasion of the intestines (including gallbladder), respiratory tract (including tonsils and adenoids), or urinary tract (if infection is present) require antibiotics to prevent spread of potential bacteria. Many physicians recommend taking antibiotics for any cuts that require stitches. We also recommend antibiotics before getting tattoos or body piercings for appropriate individuals.

On the other hand, cardiac catheterization, shedding of primary teeth, tympanostomy tube insertion, bronchoscopy, gastrointestinal endoscopy, and uncomplicated vaginal delivery and cesarean delivery do *not* necessarily require antibiotic coadministration to reduce bacterial infection.

Having More Children

Now that I've had one baby with CHD, am I at higher risk for another one?

Dr. Benson: Yes, the recurrence risk is increased. The general population risk is about 1 percent (1 in 100). If you have one baby with CHD, the risk increases to approximately 2 percent (2 in 100). The risk for a parent with CHD to have an affected offspring increases to 3 percent. If two family members are affected (parent or sibling), the risk increases to 10 percent. If there are more than two affected family members, the recurrence risk is 50 percent (even chance).

How might the information gathered during genetic counseling help me?

Dr. Benson: If a genetic cause is identified, genetic testing may lead to improved risk assessment for subsequent pregnancies.

Should I get a fetal echo when I'm pregnant with my next child? How helpful is this? What will it tell me?

Dr. Benson: A normal fetal echo done by a skilled operator with knowledge of CHD can be reassuring in assessing a "high risk" situation. In addition, if CHD is diagnosed by fetal echo, there is some benefit to being able to review the treatment options before a decision needs to be made to better plan and coordinate postnatal care. (See chapter 1 for more on fetal echocardiograms.)

Dr. Huhta: A fetal echo with the next pregnancy can be reassuring and is indicated. While a fetal echo cannot guarantee that your child will be born with a completely normal heart, in experienced hands, significant congenital heart disease can be excluded with a high confidence. A fetal echo at eighteen to twenty weeks should have a 95 percent accuracy in identifying the defect.

"Since we had lived through heart surgery and knew, though difficult, we could survive it, we opted out of the in utero cardiac sonogram. We knew we would have the baby anyway."

—*Laurie Strongin, mom to Henry (tetralogy of Fallot)*

"If I had known ahead of time that my first child was going to have CHD, it may have taken some of the joy out of that pregnancy. With the second, I was already nervous, so it was better to know as much as possible ahead of time."

—*Gerri Freid Kramer, mom to Max (tetralogy of Fallot)*

CHAPTER 8
DEALING WITH THE DIFFICULT TIMES

Betsy Adler, M.S.N., R.N., C.P.N.P.

Michael D. Freed, M.D.

James C. Huhta, M.D.

Michael J. Landzberg, M.D.

Ranae Larsen, M.D.

Peter B. Manning, M.D.

Marlon S. Rosenbaum, M.D.

Amnon Rosenthal, M.D.

Kenneth Schowengerdt, Jr., M.D.

Lisa Wispé, M.S.N., R.N., C.P.N.P.

"DIFFICULT" is a relative term. Anyone reading this book has faced difficult times, but a small group of CHD parents have faced or will face gut-wrenching, ongoing, agonizingly difficult times. Some have a child whose development has been significantly slowed or whose activities have been seriously restricted. Some have wrestled day after day with the basics—nourishing their children or finding a way to pay for all the medical bills and missed workdays. Some have a child on the list for a heart transplant. Some have watched their child have a stroke. And some have even lost a child to CHD.

As I've read through some of the things parents have written in our surveys and on the Web, I've been struck by several things. Lesson 1: The bad isn't bad all the time. CHD may always lurk in your mind, but when you manage to put it aside for minutes, hours, days, or months—and when you realize that you've done that—things become a little more bearable. Lesson 2: There is strength in numbers. As bad as it seems, you are probably not the only one who's been through whatever it is you are going through. Thanks to the Internet and to the huge number of parents who want to support other parents, you can find people to "unload" on, and it helps. And in the process, you might even learn something new that could help your child. Lesson 3: Medical advances, strength of will, and miracles can and often do prevail. Stories abound of children who have survived and thrived, despite dire predictions. Generations ago, most children born with a heart problem were sent home without any possible treatment. Today, children are being operated on before they leave the womb. How far we've come!

Our hearts go out to all of you for whom this chapter is an important one.

Gerri

When a child has no symptoms, how can you be sure that all is well?

Dr. Manning, Nurse Adler, and Nurse Wispé: Symptoms often help alert us to problems with heart function, but the lack of symptoms does not assure us that everything is well. Sometimes subtle changes that parents notice over time turn out to be very important clues that an underlying problem exists. Changes in exercise tolerance, in appetite, or in energy level are examples.

It's very important to continue recommended follow-up with your cardiologist and primary care physician because many children with heart problems may not develop symptoms until problems have advanced to the point that the heart's typically ample ability to compensate for extra work is depleted. Changes in the heart sounds on physical examination, and changes in EKGs or chest X rays can give your doctor clues about problems long before symptoms develop. Periodic echocardiograms are frequently the best sources of information about the structure and function of the heart following surgery.

Dr. Rosenthal: Subtle changes not apparent to the child, parents, or on physical examination may often be detected by noninvasive laboratory tests and occasionally require heart catheterization. With time, we get to know our children well and can recognize changes that may not be apparent to others. Continuity of care both with the primary care physician and the cardiologist may be helpful in detecting changes before symptoms appear.

By and large, if the child has no symptoms and the heart examination and the appropriate laboratory tests performed are said by the cardiologist to show no serious problem, all is indeed well.

If my child has had surgery, why are there still problems?

Dr. Freed: Some types of congenital heart disease are very complex and cannot be completely repaired by surgery. In these cases there are some residual structural abnormalities. In other instances no reparative operation is possible, and surgery can be done to improve the quality of life but not eliminate the underlying condition.

"[The hardest thing for us is] knowing that my child has a life-threatening condition with an uncertain life expectancy. We have no idea how long her heart will last—a transplant is not an option."

—*Sheryl Lamb, mom to Heather (double outlet right ventricle, hypoplastic right upper chamber, transposition, subvalvular pulmonary stenosis, bilateral superior vena cava with interrupted inferior vena cava, common ventricle)*

"Don't be complacent. Until the defect is resolved, it needs constant monitoring. If you get complacent you're going to be shocked when something goes wrong."

—*Pat Posada Klapper, mom to Alexandra (VSD)*

"Three years postsurgery, Lissie still has a small amount of leaking in her aortic and mitral valve as well as an enlarged left ventricle. They're not sure why the ventricle is larger, so all we can do is watch it and hope she grows into it. Since it doesn't appear to be affecting her at all, her doctor isn't too worried about it—for now. We'll see what the future brings."

—*Shari Maurer, mom to Lissie (tetralogy of Fallot)*

My child had surgery several weeks ago and is complaining of severe pain under her sternum. What is this a sign of, and what should we do?

Dr. Schowengerdt: Severe pain under the sternum may be musculoskeletal pain related to the trauma of the surgical incisions of the chest. However, if it's been several weeks since the operation, this is less likely to be the cause, and the situation requires prompt evaluation. Depending upon the type of heart disease that your child has, it is possible that the pain may be related to a lack of oxygen to the heart muscle, but this is uncommon. Other potential causes include an infection within the chest, fluid or infection within the sac that surrounds the heart (pericardium), or inflammation of the pericardial sac.

Why do some children have seizures and strokes after surgery? Can this cause long-term damage?

Dr. Schowengerdt: Many types of corrective surgery for congenital heart defects require the heart to be stopped while the surgeon carries out the repair. To support the circulation and supply oxygen to the other organs and tissues, children undergoing these procedures must be placed on cardiopulmonary bypass—the "heart/lung bypass machine." Because the blood must pass through this artificial system, there is a small but known risk of seizures and strokes related to microscopic blood clots or alterations in blood flow to the brain. If your child has a preexisting seizure disorder or neurologic condition, this risk may increase.

Seizures that occur in the first twenty-four to forty-eight hours after surgery, in the absence of any evident neurologic injury such as a stroke, generally do not lead to long-term effects. If a stroke were to occur, long-term effects could vary from virtually none to significant, depending upon the initial amount of injury.

Can the stitches come loose in my child's VSD repair? How will I know if this happens? Can the patch come loose? How will I know?

Dr. Schowengerdt: When a ventricular septal defect is repaired, the surgeon uses specialized material to create a "patch" that is sutured along its edges to close the defect. In rare instances, especially in the case of a defect whose location within the heart makes it difficult for the surgeon to get to, sutures may pull through some of the tissue, leading to a residual "leak" across the patch. Even if this does not occur, a tiny amount of leak may actually be seen by echocardiography in the early postoperative period. Because the leak is generally quite small, it does not allow sufficient blood flow across it to create symptoms in your child. As heart tissue grows over the patch in the several months after surgery, these small leaks generally disappear.

It is possible, but extremely unusual, for a larger portion of the patch to come loose after surgery. In this instance, since a larger amount of blood flow makes its way across the defect, your child may have symptoms and physical findings similar to those noted before the operation.

You should remember that these problems, if they occur, do so in the early postoperative period. It would be extremely unlikely for significant problems with the patch to occur after your child is discharged from the hospital and the healing process is well under way.

Can the patch or stitches in my child's heart become infected? How will I know if this has happened? What can I do to prevent this?

Dr. Manning, Nurse Adler, and Nurse Wispé: Infections of the patch or sutures in the heart are possible but very rare. A persistent fever might suggest that kind of infection. Wound infections are more common but also relatively rare after heart surgery. The best prevention is keeping the incisions clean. Wound infections are characterized by redness, swelling, pain, and/or drainage from the incision.

What is an arrhythmia?

Dr. Freed: An arrhythmia is an irregularity of the heart rate or rhythm. The irregularity may come from the top chamber of the heart (atrium) or the bottom chamber (ventricle).

Why is my child at risk for one?

Dr. Freed: Certain arrhythmias have been associated with heart disease. The arrhythmia may develop either prior to or following surgical procedures. Other types of arrhythmias aren't associated with other structural heart disease and occur in isolation.

Could my child die from an arrhythmia?

Dr. Freed: While very unusual, fatalities have been observed from arrhythmias. Your child's doctor can tell whether your child's arrhythmia is serious.

Can I do anything to prevent this?

Dr. Freed: Occasionally medicines (antiarrythmic agents) are prescribed to reduce the incidence of the arrhythmia and to prevent the more serious consequences. Unfortunately, the medications aren't always effective.

What is sudden death, and why is my child at risk for it?

Dr. Freed: Some children with very serious heart disease can have a progressively downhill course and eventually succumb to their heart disease. Occasionally the deaths are unexpected or sudden. These are almost always due to some type of arrhythmia. Your child's doctor can tell you whether your child is at any risk for sudden death.

What is bacterial endocarditis?

Dr. Rosenbaum: Bacterial endocarditis is an infection that involves a localized portion of the heart. In a typical case, bacteria enters the bloodstream from a remote part of the body, perhaps through the oral cavity or a skin infection, and becomes attached to a part of the heart—often an abnormal heart valve, an area of turbulence, or prosthetic material such as a Dacron tube. Bacterial endocarditis nearly always occurs in patients with some type of structural heart problem. The infection may damage the heart valve or the electrical system of the heart, or it may develop into a mass-like structure known as a vegetation. These vegetations may become very large and mobile. A portion of the vegetation can break off and travel to a vital organ of the body such as the brain and produce major damage.

How is bacterial endocarditis detected?

Dr. Rosenbaum: The most common symptom of bacterial endocarditis is an unexplained fever. Weight loss and night sweats are also common symptoms and are more frequent when the infection has been present for more than a few days. Blood cultures are essential to determine whether bacteria is present in the blood as well as to identify what type of organism caused the infection. The type of bacteria often determines the clinical presentation. Some bacteria cause an acute illness and often result in rapid valve destruction. Other bacteria produce a more indolent cause and result in a longer period of time before the infection is detected.

An echocardiogram is performed to localize the site of the infection and may provide information regarding heart valve involvement or the presence of vegetations. If the infection has damaged one of the heart valves such as the aortic or mitral, it frequently produces a leak in the valve or will worsen a preexisting one. The leak produces a cardiac murmur. The more severe the leak, the more likelihood there will be symptoms like shortness of breath or fluid retention.

How is bacterial endocarditis treated?

Dr. Rosenbaum: Bacterial endocarditis is treated with intravenous antibiotics, generally for four to six weeks. If the infection has caused significant valve dysfunction with congestive heart failure, cardiac surgery is often necessary to replace the valve. Surgery may also be required if the infection cannot be eradicated with antibiotics, if there has been embolization from a vegetation to a vital organ, or if there is a myocardial abscess.

Why is my child at higher risk for bacterial endocarditis?

Dr. Freed: All of us, whether or not we have heart disease, have times when bacteria can enter the blood vessels. Normally the white blood cells and antibodies remove these bacteria within a half hour or so, and no infection results. But if there's turbulence within the heart, the inner layer of the heart may be damaged slightly, and bacteria can land on the abnormal area and grow, overwhelming the body's defenses. This infection can largely be prevented by maintaining good dental hygiene and by taking antibiotics prior to any dental work involving bleeding around the gums or some surgical procedures.

Does everyone with a heart murmur need to take prophylactic antibiotics before all dental procedures and other surgeries?

Dr. Schowengerdt: Children with most forms of congenital heart disease should receive antibiotic prophylaxis to prevent the rare occurrence of endocarditis, a bacterial infection of the lining of the heart or the heart valves. Your child's cardiologist will advise you and your child as to the necessity of endocarditis prophylaxis, and, if indicated, will provide you with a wallet-size card to present to other healthcare professionals that outlines the required prophylaxis.

If a murmur is deemed to be "innocent" or "functional," no restrictions are necessary and antibiotic prophylaxis is not indicated.

What is pericarditis? How is it detected? How is it treated?

Dr. Rosenbaum: The heart is enclosed in a sac known as the pericardium. Pericarditis refers to inflammation of the pericardium from any one of a number of causes. In the vast majority of cases, the cause is unknown and presumed to be viral. Sometimes pericarditis occurs after cardiac surgery and is known as postpericardiotomy syndrome, or PPS. Pericarditis may also develop as a result of an autoimmune disorder, such as lupus erythematosus. In rare instances, it may complicate a bacterial infection or a malignancy.

Pericarditis typically produces fluid accumulation within the pericardial sac. It often results in a sharp chest pain that may radiate into the shoulder. The pain is worse when breathing in and is usually improved by sitting forward. Fever may also be present. Examination typically reveals a pericardial rub. When these findings are present, an echocardiogram is performed to confirm the diagnosis by assessing whether there is fluid in the pericardium.

Most forms of pericarditis are treated with anti-inflammatory medications that include aspirin, non-steroidal anti-inflammatory agents such as indocin or Motrin, and corticosteroids. These medications provide pain relief and decrease the inflammation around the heart. Most forms of pericarditis resolve over time, although recurrences are possible. In rare instances, pericarditis becomes chronic and produces constriction around the heart. Those patients may require surgery to remove the pericardium.

What is viral myocarditis?

Dr. Rosenbaum: Myocarditis is a general term applied to inflammation involving the heart muscle. Viral myocarditis may be caused by certain common viruses that can affect the heart muscle. The clinical manifestations are extremely variable. Mild cases may not even be recognized and resolve spontaneously. More severe cases cause impairment of heart muscle function and may produce symptoms including shortness of breath, fluid accumulation, and/or rhythm abnormalities.

Once myocarditis is present, the subsequent course is variable. Some cases may resolve completely, others evolve into a dilated cardiomyopathy over time, and a subset develop a rapid downhill course in which heart transplantation is the only option.

How is viral myocarditis detected?

Dr. Rosenbaum: The diagnosis of myocarditis is usually made only after a patient develops symptoms related to heart muscle dysfunction (such as shortness of breath or fluid retention) or arrhythmias (such as palpitations, dizziness, or heart racing). Chest pain is less common but may occur if the pericardium is involved. An echocardiogram provides a noninvasive and accurate assessment of the heart muscle chamber size and function.

How is viral myocarditis treated?

Dr. Rosenbaum: Viral myocarditis is treated with medications that improve cardiac output and arrhythmias, if present. The specific virus is not usually identified. Treatment depends on the extent of heart muscle impairment and symptoms. Patients with impaired cardiac function and shortness of breath are treated with an ACE inhibitor, a diuretic, and digoxin. An ACE inhibitor lowers the blood pressure and improves cardiac output. A diuretic helps to eliminate excess fluid. Digoxin enhances cardiac muscle contraction and can be useful in treating rhythm problems that originate from the top of the heart. Patients with the most severe forms of myocarditis require hospitalization and treatment with intravenous medications or mechanical support to augment heart muscle function. Some of these patients may require heart transplantation.

What is cardiomyopathy? How is it detected? How is it treated?

Dr. Rosenbaum: Cardiomyopathy is a general term that refers to abnormalities of the heart muscle. Cardiomyopathy is frequently classified into three different categories: dilated, hypertrophic, and restrictive.

Dilated cardiomyopathy is characterized by enlargement of the cardiac chambers and impaired heart muscle function. There are many potential causes of dilated cardiomyopathy, including infection (such as viral myocarditis), toxin-induced (such as by alcohol), metabolic, immunologic, and familial. In most cases, the exact cause cannot be identified and is referred to as idiopathic.

The diagnosis of dilated cardiomyopathy is typically made because the patient has developed cardiac symptoms such as shortness of breath, fluid retention, or heart rhythm abnormalities. The diagnosis is confirmed with an echocardiogram. This test is noninvasive and accurately assesses the cardiac chamber size and thickness, heart muscle function, and any associated valve abnormalities.

Patients with symptoms generally have progressive deterioration over time. Treatment for dilated cardiomyopathy will depend on the symptoms and severity. Most patients are treated with an ACE inhibitor, which improves cardiac output. Patients with fluid retention or symptoms of shortness of breath are also treated with a diuretic, as well as digoxin, which augments heart muscle contraction and is useful for treatment of atrial arrhythmias. In addition, some patients benefit from the addition of a beta-blocker.

Patients with dilated cardiomyopathy may also experience atrial and ventricular arrhythmias and may require specific treatment for these problems. Patients with the most severe forms of dilated cardiomyopathy may require hospitalization to receive intravenous medications as well as evaluation for heart transplantation.

Hypertrophic cardiomyopathy is a form of congenital heart disease characterized by the presence of an inappropriately thick heart muscle. This abnormality occurs in several different patterns. The excess thickness may involve a part or all of the left ventricle. In some cases, the ventricular septum is particularly thick just below the aortic valve. This form of hypertrophic cardiomyopathy is also referred to as idiopathic hypertrophic subaortic stenosis. The disorder can occasionally involve the right ventricle. Hypertrophic cardiomyopathy is genetically transmitted as an autosomal dominant trait in 50 percent of cases. However, there is considerable variability in the manifestations of this disease among family members who have inherited this trait. Some may have mild abnormalities, while others may have a more pronounced form. The remaining 50 percent of hypertrophic cardiomyopathy cases occur throughout the population without any family history of the disorder.

HCM may not produce symptoms when it is mild, but more typically it results in chest pain, shortness of breath, fainting spells, or rhythm problems. Unfortunately, sudden death may be the first clinical manifestation of this disorder.

The treatment of hypertrophic cardiomyopathy will depend on both symptoms and anatomic issues. Patients with no cardiac symptoms may not even know they have this disorder. Symptoms such as shortness of breath or chest pain can usually be effectively treated with a beta-blocker or a calcium channel blocker. Once the diagnosis is made, patients are advised against strenuous exercise.

When the ventricular septum is markedly thick just under the aortic valve, it can produce obstruction to blood flow and contribute to the symptoms of shortness of breath, chest pain, or dizziness. When medications are not effective, or when the obstruction is particularly severe, cardiac surgery can be performed to remove the excess muscle. This procedure is known as a septal myotomy or myomectomy. In some cases, a permanent pacemaker has been effective in reducing the degree of obstruction and improving symptoms. Recently, a procedure known as alcohol ablation has been employed to occlude the blood supply to the septal artery of the heart. This procedure causes localized damage to the muscle of the ventricular septum at the site of the obstruction. There is currently not enough information to assess the potential role of this procedure in the treatment of this disease.

Restrictive cardiomyopathy is an unusual form of heart disease. It is characterized by an excessively stiff heart muscle that abnormally fills the ventricle. As a result, patients frequently complain of exercise intolerance, weakness, and shortness of breath. There are many causes of a restrictive cardiomyopathy; it may be the result of myocardial disease, infiltration of the myocardium by abnormal substances, or inherited disorders. The treatment varies with the specific cause.

What is mitral valve prolapse? How is it detected? How is it treated?

Dr. Rosenbaum: Mitral valve prolapse is a very common disorder that occurs in 3 to 5 percent of the population. It is more frequently seen in women. While the disorder usually occurs as an isolated entity, it may sometimes be part of a more generalized disorder such as Marfan's syndrome or Ehlers-Danlos syndrome. Mitral valve prolapse seems to occur more frequently in patients with an asthenic build—those with a straight back, or pectus excavatum.

In some cases, mitral valve prolapse consists of a slight exaggeration in the normal billowing of the mitral valve leaflets into the left atrium whereas in other cases, the abnormality is more pronounced and results in a leak in the mitral valve (mitral regurgitation). The mitral valve leaflets may also be referred to as "redundant" or "floppy."

The clinical findings in patients with mitral valve prolapse are quite variable. While most patients are asymptomatic, some patients may complain of dizziness, palpitations, chest discomfort, or diminished exercise capacity when a significant degree of mitral regurgitation is present. Other symptoms that can be difficult to relate to the mitral valve prolapse include fatigue and a variety of neuropsychiatric symptoms. The findings on physical examination may vary over time and can include the presence of a "midsystolic click" and mitral regurgitation.

It is important to emphasize that some patients may be diagnosed with mitral valve prolapse on the basis of an echocardiogram in the absence of symptoms or abnormalities on examination. Since there may be overlap between a normal mitral valve and mild prolapse on an echocardiogram, the potential for overdiagnosis of this entity does exist.

Patients with chest pain or palpitation are often treated with a beta-blocker. Antibiotic prophylaxis against bacterial endocarditis is recommended for certain groups of patients with mitral valve prolapse. Patients with an important degree of mitral regurgitation are candidates for mitral valve repair or replacement.

What is atrial tachycardia, and why does it occur? Can I do anything to prevent it?

Dr. Schowengerdt: A fast heart rate is referred to as tachycardia. The most common type of abnormal tachycardia is atrial tachycardia, meaning that the fast heart rate originates in the upper chambers of the heart (the atria) or the upper portion of the cardiac conduction system. There are several types of atrial tachycardia, which may be caused by an area of abnormal tissue within the atrial muscle itself or by the presence of an abnormal pathway of the specialized conduction tissue of the heart.

Occasionally, atrial tachycardia may occur after your child's heart operation as a result of either his preexisting heart condition or related to the surgery involving the atrial tissue.

In many instances, medications are required to control the tachycardia and prevent its recurrence. If this is the case, it's important for your child to take the prescribed medication regularly as directed to prevent potential recurrences.

In older children with significant episodes of certain types of atrial tachycardia, specialized testing requiring a cardiac catheterization may identify the cause of the tachycardia, and eliminating the abnormal area within the heart using a catheter technique called radio-frequency ablation may prevent its recurrence. Radio-frequency ablation applies very localized energy to the inner surface of the heart to eliminate the abnormal conduction tissue.

What is heart block, and how is it treated?

Dr. Schowengerdt: Heart block refers to several types of conditions that involve a failure of the heart's electrical impulses to pass in a normal manner through its conduction system from the upper chambers (atria) to the lower chambers (the ventricles). Heart block may be present at birth (congenital), or may occur as an unavoidable complication of heart surgery, as the conduction system may pass very close to the defects being repaired. One of the most significant forms of heart block is referred to as complete heart block, when the atria and the ventricles beat independently at their own respective rates. Because the rate of contraction of the ventricular muscle itself, without stimulation from the normal conduction pathway, may be excessively slow, your child may require an artificial pacemaker.

In this situation, wires to stimulate the heart to beat when necessary are attached to the heart wall, and are connected to a very small (approximately two inches in diameter) control and battery unit. This pacemaker is placed under the skin of the abdomen or the chest wall.

"I've been told no monkey bars, no pickup under the armpits, no microwave, no magnet right here [pointing to chest] unless my mom's checking my pacemaker. It's scary going in if you've never had heart surgery before. After that it's pretty cool, especially in camp."

—*Eileen Garcia, nine years old (symptomatic bradycardia,*
second-degree heart block with a pacemaker,
Edward Madden Open Hearts Camp camper)

What is sick sinus syndrome? How is it detected? How is it treated?

Dr. Schowengerdt: The sinus node, or pacemaker of the heart, is normally in the right atrium and functions to initiate each heartbeat. If the sinus node is diseased, it may not function properly, and sick sinus syndrome may result. In this case, if no other region of the heart is able to control the heart rate appropriately, the heart rate may become abnormally slow, and symptoms may result. These symptoms relate to impaired output of blood to the body and may include restless sleep, excessive fatigue, dizziness, or fainting episodes. Sick sinus syndrome may be detected on a prolonged EKG tracing or by a special monitor. Sick sinus syndrome is unusual in children but if present may require treatment with an artificial pacemaker.

My child needs a pacemaker. How is it put in and by whom?

Dr. Huhta: A pediatric heart surgeon or a pediatric cardiologist will place the pacemaker in the chest or under the skin depending on the size of the child and the type of pacing required.

Will he feel the pacemaker while it is in?

Dr. Huhta: The pacing beats should not cause any sensation if the pacemaker is properly adjusted.

How would we know if it stopped working?

Dr. Huhta: Regular pacemaker checks are routine, and you may receive a machine to send pacemaker recordings over the telephone regularly.

My child was repaired as a baby, but he's ten now and the doctors have told us that he needs a new valve. What causes this?

Dr. Huhta: The valve doesn't grow with your child, so if a valve was placed in your baby and the child has since grown five to ten times in weight, then the valve will have to be replaced.

Why does a valve problem occur after a repair?

Dr. Huhta: Valves are foreign material, and the body will slowly reject anything foreign. This slow immunological process causes deterioration of the valve and accelerates the natural aging process, causing the valve either to leak or to become narrowed.

How do we know when it is time for a transplant?

Dr. Larsen: Most children undergo successful repair of their congenital heart disease and don't ever need cardiac transplantation. Occasionally, usually because of the development of poor function of the heart muscle unresponsive to medicines, replacement of the heart is needed. In this situation your cardiologist may want to consider transplantation when your child can't tolerate exercise or participate in normal activities such as school, or if your child develops a significant risk of sudden death. Although cardiac transplantation is generally reserved for children in whom no other options exist, significant strides have been made during the past decade in the transplantation of hearts in children with congenital heart disease. Transplantation can now offer hope to some children with severe heart disease who previously died from their condition.

Dr. Schowengerdt: In some children, such as those with severe heart muscle disease (cardiomyopathy) or those with complex heart defects for which further conventional surgical therapies are not possible and life expectancy is severely limited, a heart transplant may be an option. Evaluation and consideration of a heart transplant is a complex and emotional situation and must be discussed fully among you, your child, and the transplant physicians and nurses. Cardiac transplantation now provides a nearly normal quality of life for adults and children for whom no other treatment options previously existed. It must be realized, however, that after a heart transplant, frequent visits to the cardiologist are necessary, medications to prevent rejection of the new heart are required throughout life, and the long-term outlook remains uncertain. The risks of developing serious infections as well as rejection of the new heart are ever-present, but become less with time. There are also other long-term problems that can occur after a heart transplant that your physician will discuss with you and your child.

If your physicians have determined that transplantation is your child's best hope of survival, if it is medically and surgically possible, and if you and your child wish to proceed, a complete transplant evaluation will be carried out. Because of the nationwide shortage of donor organs, once the decision is made that transplantation is necessary and possible, your child will be placed on the national waiting list as soon as possible. The urgency of proceeding to the actual transplant will depend upon your cardiologist's assessment of your child's current condition. Children who are critically ill are treated in the hospital until a suitable donor organ is available for transplantation. Children who are more stable may remain at home while awaiting a transplant.

"Our son had a surgery at four days and a surgery at three months, which were steps that needed to be taken before correction surgery. The correction surgery took place around eighteen months, but because scar tissue developed, there was more to do than they expected. They couldn't finish the correction and so another surgery had to be done. That open-heart surgery happened when he was close to two and a half, but after one year's time, his body was "calcifying" the new pulmonary artery that they gave him. This happens to some children, but not all. They ballooned it open and placed a stent. This held him for approximately ten months before they did another open-heart surgery at about four and a half years.

"Without more detail, the point is: There can be complications, and there are no guarantees. How do you face this? You don't, and you dread future appointments because you're never sure what you'll find out next.

"It is so important that once you leave the doctor's office or hospital, you enjoy your days together. Plan fun things. Enjoy a normal life and take the rest as it comes. When it comes, you'll get through it again and then continue on enjoying your family and the blessings that God gives you."

—Sharon Popp, mom to Ben
(pulmonary atresia with VSD, transposition of the aorta)

"What happened in surgery was that they had nicked a few thin veins that carry the fatty fluids from the foods she ate. But no one told us that [in her case] Alyssa was supposed to eat nonfat foods for a few weeks after surgery so that she could heal. As a result she got chylothorax and fluid accumulated in front of her lungs that had to be drained out."

—Michelle Goenner, mom to Alyssa Mae
(dextrocardia, heterotaxy asplenic syndrome,
double outlet right ventricle, severe pulmonary stenosis)

CHAPTER 9
GROWING UP

Betsy Adler, M.S.N., R.N., C.P.N.P.   Peter B. Manning, M.D.
Jonas I. Bromberg, Psy.D.   Marlon Rosenbaum, M.D.
Michael J. Landzberg, M.D.   Lisa Wispé, M.S.N., R.N., C.P.N.P.

Some of our readers have children who are nearing their teen years, but for those of you who are the parents of newborns, adolescence and adulthood may seem an unimaginable distance in the future. However, we felt it was important to look forward to get a glimpse of what may lie ahead. I know that as a mother of a little girl, one of my main concerns was whether Lissie's heart defect would affect her ability to have children.

We also had the opportunity to get input from adults who were born with some form of CHD. We thought it would be helpful to hear their thoughts on what it's like living with CHD. An important thing to bear in mind when reading about adults with CHD is that repairs are done a lot differently today than they were several years ago, so life expectancies and quality-of-life issues can be different. We don't really know how the children who are repaired today will do (though my guess is that they will be doing even better than those who were repaired twenty years ago) or what technology will arise to improve things even more for our children.

Shari

"Take it from someone who has been through it all, too. [Your child with CHD] won't remember the first two years, maybe even three or four. Two of my first memories of my CHD are being a tester for echos and the transistor they used pinching me. I was somewhere between four and five. The other is being in the hospital for bacterial endocarditis when I was five. I was in the hospital for thirty-two days on IV antibiotics. I only have good memories of that stay. It was time I got to spend with my daddy, because he stayed *every* night, and got up early and went to work the next morning. I do remember the IV sticks, blood draws . . . but they don't stand out as much as the play-room, the wagon rides in the hall, the time I took a bath and purposely wet my IV so they would take it out, and it worked, at least for the time I was in the tub.

"I feel I am who I am because of my CHD. Fighting for my life taught me how to live and enjoy life to its fullest, and not take *anything* for granted."

—Laura Wade, twenty-nine-year-old ACHDer
(*single ventricle, transposition of the great vessels, pulmonary atresia*)

Approaching Adulthood

Does puberty have any special effect on CHD?

Dr. Landzberg: The simple answer is "Absolutely!!" The effects include medical changes such as:

- rapid growth spurts with increasing demands on heart, lung, muscle, and skeletal function;
- hormonal fluxes that affect breathing pattern, muscle, fat and water distribution, and bone growth;
- onset of menarche, with potential shifts in iron levels and blood counts.

In addition, issues involved with emotional development may also appear at this time, including self-esteem, independence, responsibility, sexuality, community, and socialization.

Who will care for my adult child?

Dr. Landzberg: The past several decades have witnessed the develop-ment of physicians, nurses, physician-assistants and other medical care-givers with unique training in the long-term coordinated care of young and older adults with congenital heart defects. Such individuals have achieved this expertise through unique training programs, incorporating pediatric, adolescent and adult expertise. Regional "centers of excellence" in the management of young and older adults with congenital heart disease are now recognized in all parts of the United States and throughout the world, with a growing network of communication amongst themselves and with local centers of expertise. Nearly all people with congenital heart disease should have both a regional and local center of expertise familiar with them and coordinated in their care.

What kind of long-term study results have been done on the life span of people with CHD?

Dr. Manning, Nurse Adler, and Nurse Wispé: Because the first open-heart surgery of any kind was performed in the 1950s, and the field has undergone considerable evolution since that time, the information on life span of people with some forms of repaired congenital heart disease is very limited. Certain defects, such as isolated atrial or ventricular septal defects in which the heart is anatomically and functionally completely normal after successful repair, should be associated with a normal life span. In any defect where there is some residual abnormality of the heart, long-term follow-up by a cardiologist is essential, and later problems may be possible.

Sex and Reproduction

Will my child be able to have sex when he is older?

Dr. Landzberg: Despite the increased demands placed upon the heart and lungs during sexual activity, I am unaware of any particular form of CHD that places an individual at acute risk from sex that does not unduly exhaust that particular individual. In other words, be smart. Have sex, but not to the point of exhaustion.

Can my daughter get pregnant when she's older?

Dr. Landzberg: Specialists guiding young and older persons with CHD can help maximize the potential for safe and successful childbearing and child rearing. They emphasize planned parenthood and the need to fully understand the acute risks to mother, father, and child well in advance of contemplating pregnancy.

Almost no prospective mothers (with the exception of those with heart failure, pulmonary hypertension, severe cyanosis, unprotected life-threatening arrhythmias, and severe uncorrected obstructive heart valve defects) are counseled to avoid pregnancy, but all should be counseled in general. Individual needs should be addressed by a combined patient–internal medicine–nursing–cardiology–obstetrics–anesthesia team, as needed, with flexible recommendations understood and agreed upon by all well in advance of anticipated pregnancy. A continued partnership with medical caregivers is a requisite for a successful pregnancy.

Are there any special needs or concerns that a pregnant woman with CHD should be aware of?

Dr. Landzberg: From its onset, pregnancy induces hormonal changes that promote water retention, abnormal changes in heart rate, filling and pumping ability, increase in extra abnormal heartbeats (arrhythmia tendency), increase in breathing pattern and inefficiency, musculoskeletal instability, change in potential iron balance and blood counts, and abnormal breakdown and use of previously stable medications. All of these factors contribute to increased fatigue and may lead to increased risk for individuals. Being pregnant with twins (or more) may exaggerate these changes. Means of delivery (vaginal vs. cesarean) should be based on the needs of mother and doctor, with intense planning and discussion beforehand and also a readiness to alter the planned approach if needed. Women who have holes in their heart need filters placed on their IVs to eliminate the possibility of an air bubble reaching the brain or other vital organs. Similarly, women with cyanosis may require oxygen during pregnancy or delivery.

Treatment of mothers who use anticoagulants ("blood thinners") before, during, and after pregnancy is intense and carries particular risks. Pregnancy carries its own tendency to promote clotting, and types and doses of medications taken to protect mothers from development of valve dysfunction, stroke, or blood clots may change at varying times during pregnancy. Frequent follow-up is essential.

What if she needs medications? Can this affect her baby?

Dr. Landzberg: Even the simplest of over-the-counter medications can be harmful to either mother or child during pregnancy, and all should be discussed during planning. Safety of the mother is always considered paramount. Almost all medications known to be threatening to the growing child have at least temporary substitutes that can be utilized during pregnancy if sufficient planning is undertaken before getting pregnant.

Should she see a "high risk" obstetrician?

Dr. Landzberg: Most regional and local centers of expertise in the care of adult patients with CHD have dedicated obstetrical subspecialists who counsel and guide prospective parents. The majority of women with CHD may not require a "high risk" scenario. "High risk" does not denote an urgent or emergent situation, but rather alerts the caregiving team to the potential for such. Levels of risk may vary within a particular pregnancy or with subsequent pregnancies.

Should she get antibiotics during pregnancy?

Dr. Landzberg: Uncomplicated vaginal or cesarean deliveries do not necessarily require antibiotics. However, antibiotics will be administered if delivery occurs while the mother has an associated infection or significant potential for developing one.

Will my daughter be able to take birth control pills?

Dr. Landzberg: Planning for parenthood is a necessary part of successful parental life and childbirth for persons with CHD. There are essentially no modern comparisons of risk and safety among the various forms of contraception. Until further studies are undertaken, recommendations should be individualized, though they may vary from institution to institution. However, there is one common recommendation: Parenthood should be planned, and contraception should be utilized.

What are my child's chances of having a baby with CHD?

Dr. Landzberg: In general, risk of your child with CHD having a baby with CHD falls between 3 and 10 percent. For unclear reasons, women with CHD tend to fall on the higher end of this risk profile. So do parents with congenital obstruction of structures on the left side of the heart, "conotruncal abnormalities" (tetralogy of Fallot, truncus arteriosus, interrupted aortic arch syndromes, and certain types of ventricular septal defects), other noncardiac genetic issues, or relatives with recognized congenital abnormalities. Genetic screening and counseling by appropriately trained caregivers may be warranted for any potential parent with CHD, but are particularly useful for parents with at least one or more recognized risks. Fetal sonography is especially useful in prenatal diagnosis and counseling.

Should my daughter (or daughter-in-law) have a fetal echo when she's pregnant?

Dr. Landzberg: While there are limitations, fetal echocardiography can help to diagnose CHD, allowing for parental planning regarding maintenance of pregnancy and promoting the ability of pediatric caregivers to provide for a safe delivery and early childhood. Fetal echocardiography is routinely performed from a transabdominal approach, optimally near the twentieth week of gestation, though it may be performed earlier in some centers transvaginally. Repeated testing may be suggested based upon findings.

Psychosocial Aspects of Growing Up with CHD

What difficulties and challenges have your patients encountered during the transition from adolescence to young adulthood?

Dr. Bromberg: (1) Uncertainty—the challenge of living a full life while not being able to count on good physical health; (2) social connectedness—the challenge of "fitting in" and avoiding social isolation due to feeling "different"; (3) health management—the challenge of learning health-enhancing and self-care skills and assuming a full role as a partner in one's health care; (4) disclosure—the challenge of learning how much information to give and to whom about one's health status; and (5) autonomy—the challenge of finding a comfortable balance between independence and dependence on others.

What can parents do while their children are still young that will help them grow into adulthood with CHD more easily?

Dr. Bromberg: My advice to parents of children with CHD is that you find medical providers who understand and take seriously the social and emotional aspects of your child's health, not just the health of his or her heart.

Help your children learn that coping with the emotional and interpersonal aspects of CHD are as important as attending to physical health issues. Talk with them about their experience of having CHD, what it makes them think about, or how it makes them feel. Set an example by talking about your own thoughts and feelings while respecting appropriate parent-child boundaries. Give them explicit permission to talk about their illness-related thoughts and feelings. Coping with the psychosocial aspects of medical illness can help children feel a sense of self-efficacy and mastery that they can apply to many other areas of life.

Seek clinical treatment programs that offer psychosocial support services. Programs that incorporate the services of a clinical social worker or clinical psychologist into their multidisciplinary treatment team show their commitment to this more holistic perspective on health.

Learn to back off when your child needs space. Learn to read your child's cues. The child's need for space can arise at any age and be motivated by many causes (even ones we might not see as logical in our adult minds). Never pressure a child to talk about his or her feelings about the illness, but always send a message that leaves the door open for a future discussion.

How can my child benefit from developing relationships with other children with CHD?

Dr. Bromberg: A consistent theme that I have heard in my discussions with adults with CHD (ACHDers) is their sense of isolation, especially as children, from others who were "like them." Younger children aren't likely to be able to observe and express their feelings about being different. Some may even insist they don't feel different, in spite of what you may observe. As children mature into young adulthood, they become better at recognizing and acknowledging these feelings. I have been impressed by the numbers of patients who report that they have never met someone else with CHD. Almost every ACHDer I have talked with has reported that meeting someone else with CHD helped them to feel as if they were not "the only one out there." Meeting others with CHD appears to facilitate a sense of community and belonging.

I have talked with many parents who have been hesitant to do this because they wanted to avoid the "complications" of having their child form a relationship with another child who might be sicker than theirs or even die at a young age. "I don't want to worry him, it will just make him think he could be that sick" and "I don't want her to think she could die" are common excuses parents make for avoiding these relationships. The "complexities" of these relationships and the potential for difficult emotions to arise should not be avoided out of fear. Instead, the opportunity should be welcomed as a chance to help your child learn to manage difficult emotions and even grow from the experience. These relationships are also important for children as another way to promote normalcy and mastery in the context of lifelong illness.

What kinds of things do you hear in patient support groups?

Dr. Bromberg: A wide range of topics are discussed in patient support groups. Discussions often focus on relationships and communication with health care providers, frustrations with the health care and insurance systems, work and family issues, and "sharing and comparing" information and experiences with various doctors, therapies, medications, procedures, and symptoms. A good deal of time is spent socializing and building community. Participants share personal and family news. New jobs, promotions, graduations, birthdays, weddings, births, and deaths are often shared with the group.

What kind of psychosocial support services do you think should be offered to ACHDers?

Dr. Bromberg: The supportive services that can be provided by a medical social worker or psychologist are most important. Psychosocial support services can be divided into four primary domains: (1) direct support, (2) information and self-care support, (3) behavior and lifestyle change, and (4) assessment and treatment of other psychological problems. The integration of these services with regular medical care can improve adaptation and coping and lead to better health outcomes.

What do you mean by direct support?

Dr. Bromberg: Direct support includes helping patients explore and cope with the emotions related to their cardiac health. Helping patients with problems such as preparation for surgery, vocational and social issues, and other interpersonal issues falls within this domain. Helping patients learn to communicate about their illness with family and friends, coworkers, and medical professionals is a form of direct support. Even those ACHDers who have adequate social support report feeling different from others in many ways, which sometimes serves as a barrier to asking for support. The feeling of "being different" can lead to a range of negative feelings, including isolation, sadness, and fear.

Individuals with CHD who do not demonstrate psychosocial adjustment difficulties may still be at risk for problems such as depression, fear, and anxiety. This risk can be reduced through direct support that acknowledges the normalcy of these feelings and openly discusses them. It is important to help patients understand that experiencing these feelings in and of itself is not an indication of an emotional problem; rather, in many cases it can be seen as a normal response to illness. Direct support also can serve as a forum to teach people skills to prevent the onset of psychosocial difficulties.

Children and adolescents are often unable or unwilling to talk about feelings related to their illness. Many of the adults I've worked with talk about having these feelings, but also feeling like they didn't want to burden their family and friends by talking about it. Children and adolescents should be given permission to talk about the emotional consequences of their illness, encouraged to view these feelings as normal, but never pressured to talk if they are not ready or willing.

Direct support also can mean direct intervention with the medical team. Helping the medical team members understand their patients' emotional lives can help medical providers gather information more effectively and conduct treatment planning and intervention in ways that are respectful of patients' individual differences and the nuances of their social contexts.

What does information and self-care support involve?

Dr. Bromberg: Information and self-care support includes helping patients learn skills to obtain important medical information and help them acquire skills to engage in appropriate self-care.

Learning to use medical terminology is important in understanding and participating in medical discussions, decision-making, and treatment planning with providers. While it may seem intimidating at first, using medical terminology makes sense for several reasons. First, a good facility with medical terms can help establish rapport with medical providers, who may view you as a more credible partner in care. Second, using medical terms can provide a bit of emotional distance, which may be useful in helping you discuss health issues more objectively and unemotionally. Finally, medical terminology is very precise and can help your provider understand you better. Knowing how to obtain and use medical information puts the patient on the inside, and allows patients the opportunity to be part of the process, rather than a passive recipient of healthcare services.

One young woman I consulted told me a story about her frustration in being unable to talk with her cardiologist about appropriate methods of contraception. Her difficulty appeared to have little to do with any embarrassment about discussing sex-related issues with her cardiologist, but rather a lack of experience in conducting any kind of direct questioning of her cardiologist because of her dependence on her parents in this role. This resulted in the woman potentially being exposed to increased cardiac risk due to her decision to use birth control pills without proper medical advice.

Structured patient education, beginning at an early age, can improve patients' understanding and lead to greater participation in their care, greater feelings of self-efficacy, and potentially improved medical outcomes. While there needs to be some balance between a child's cognitive and emotional levels of development and the information they are given, even very young children can learn the basic language to communicate about their heart anatomy, diagnosis, and corrective procedures. Providing accurate language for children facilitates their ability to obtain social support and play an active role in their care. Teaching young children medical terminology also helps to demystify the world of their illness and may help prevent misconceptions and fears from arising.

Children who participate as partners in their care are often more cooperative with medical recommendations and treatments and are more likely to form trusting relationships with their providers. Parents should encourage medical providers to speak directly to their children rather than allowing them to just converse with the parent. There will be times when it might be appropriate for your medical providers to speak directly to you, without your child present. In some cases it might be better to schedule these discussions at a separate time when your child is not present. Leaving children out of medical discussions, either by not inviting them in or asking them to leave the room, may raise a child's anxiety significantly. Children often make up fantasies about these private conversations that can be far worse than what they might actually hear.

Patients feel empowered by the increased sense of control that comes with learning appropriate self-care: how to assess which symptoms and circumstances require professional attention and how to take care of the rest themselves.

People coping with lifelong illness should complete an inventory of their social support network at various stages of development, as life evolves and support resources change. In the beginning you can do this for yourself, on your child's behalf; in time you can explain and he or she can contribute, and you can teach strategies you have developed for engaging support. Even very young children can think about people they like to talk with about health-related issues.

How do you work with patients on behavioral and lifestyle changes?

Dr. Bromberg: Psychosocial services aim to help patients identify behavior patterns that impact disease, such as diet, alcohol use, smoking, and physical activity. Following the identification of such behaviors, the second step is to help patients make adjustments and changes in lifestyle that reduce their cardiac risk and enhance their health. Systematic efforts at behavior change often work better than informal efforts, so engaging the support of a behavioral change specialist in making necessary changes can be very helpful.

Even though stress is more commonly thought of as a detrimental influence in relation to acquired heart disease, it also plays a critical role in the health of congenital heart patients. It is important to address stress, as it may lead a patient to return to anxiety-reducing behaviors such as smoking or overeating. Learning healthy ways to reduce stress supports behavior change and reduces stress-related symptoms. Medical difficulties can themselves produce heightened states of sympathetic nervous system arousal (i.e., "stress"), which can have a detrimental long-term effect on emotional well-being and physiological functioning. Research has demonstrated that in some cases relaxation can mediate such problems as high blood pressure, arrhythmia, and insomnia.

Insight from an Adult CHD Specialist (Marlon S. Rosenbaum, M.D.)

When our children were diagnosed with CHD, there was a lot of "here and now" to deal with—looking at the anatomy of the heart, watching falling blood oxygen levels, thinking about pending surgery. But when the day was over, we would lay awake wondering about the future. We wanted to talk to a seven-year-old and a twenty-seven-year-old to find out how CHD affected their everyday lives. And we wanted to know if CHD would affect our children's lifespan. We weren't alone. When we surveyed parents, the lifespan question in particular came up over and over.

These are questions that can't be answered definitively. Every case is different. Technology has changed dramatically over the last few decades and continues to advance. Still, we thought it would be nice to end this book with a look at what we can learn from the past and expect from the future.

Gerri and Shari

Can you tell us some success stories you've seen during your practice?

Dr. Rosenbaum: Several years ago, a colleague referred a young man with complex cyanotic congenital heart disease to me. This twenty-six-year-old man had undergone two palliative operations in the past to improve his oxygen level, but corrective surgery was considered too risky. The second operation did not improve his situation and his recovery from that operation had been difficult. His oxygen level became extremely low and he was not able to climb more than a few steps before becoming short of breath.

When I met the family, they were extremely apprehensive and reluctant to discuss another operation, especially one that was risky. We performed a cardiac catheterization, which demonstrated that cardiac surgery was feasible but very complicated. Surgery was finally scheduled, but the day before the operation the family wanted to cancel it. Although the parents understood how severely limited their son was, they were frightened by the possibility of a bad outcome. They wanted to be reassured that everything would be fine. This was a difficult situation for me. I knew that this would be a complicated operation that if successful, would dramatically improve this patient's life. I carefully urged the family to proceed with the operation.

The operation was very long and difficult. It required the reconstruction of the only remaining pulmonary artery, removal of a shunt, insertion of a conduit between the ventricle and the pulmonary artery, and closure of a very large VSD.

The operation was successful. The patient is no longer short of breath or cyanotic and he is now able to exercise normally.

Eight years ago, I saw a sixty-six-year-old man with tetralogy of Fallot. The patient had undergone a Brock procedure in 1953 in an attempt to increase blood flow to the lungs by stretching open a narrowed pulmonary valve. This palliative procedure was tried before corrective surgery was possible. For unknown reasons, this patient was never referred for corrective surgery.

We repaired his congenital heart disease. The operation was straight-forward and his postoperative course was uncomplicated. The patient wrote me one year later describing how much his life had changed. He was exercising three times a week and wished that he had known about this surgery years before.

Five years ago, I evaluated a college student who had just been diag-nosed with Ebstein's anomaly. The patient was born prematurely and had chronic symptoms of shortness of breath with very limited activity. Her symptoms had been attributed to lung problems related to either asthma or her prematurity. She was seen at her college infirmary because of fever and was found to have an elevated red blood cell count. A cardiac echo showed Ebstein's anomaly and a hole in the upper chamber (ASD) that allowed blood to bypass the lungs, and enter the arterial circulation without receiv-ing oxygen. This was producing cyanosis and shortness of breath. With ex-ercise, more and more blood would traverse the hole in the atrium, bypass the lungs, and produce more cyanosis. Surgery was performed to correct the Ebstein's anomaly and close the ASD. After the operation, her cyanosis was eliminated and her exercise capacity improved dramatically.

In general, how has the treatment of and prognosis for congenital heart defects changed over the years?

Dr. Rosenbaum: There have been steady improvements in the treat-ment of congenital heart disease since the development of cardiac surgery. The first cardiac operations were performed in patients with relatively simple cardiac abnormalities, such as atrial septal defect, ventricular sep-tal defect, aortic stenosis, pulmonic stenosis, and tetralogy of Fallot. In-fants were treated with palliative procedures, such as shunts or pulmonary artery banding, but cardiac repair early in life was very high risk. Over the past two decades, improvements in both the medical and surgical manage-ment have enabled physicians at experienced centers to repair complex defects during infancy with very low risk. Surgical complications have di-minished considerably.

The long-term results of the operations performed several decades ago allowed us to modify current approaches to improve upon the results of the early operations. The prognosis has improved for the vast majority of these defects. Before the development of cardiac surgery, many children with congenital heart disease did not reach adulthood. Some patients underwent palliative procedures, which delayed the need for corrective surgery but oc-casionally caused irreversible damage to the pulmonary arteries.

So much has now changed. Improvements in myocardial protec-tion during cardiac surgery have led to better heart muscle function after surgery. Serious cardiac rhythm problems are now more effectively treated. Many of the severe defects that could not be repaired during the 1970s and 1980s can now be treated surgically. Finally, patients with hearts that cannot be repaired can usually be offered heart transplantation.

If I have a young child or infant who has just been diagnosed with CHD, what can I learn from an adult who was diagnosed with CHD thirty or more years ago?

Dr. Rosenbaum: The adult who underwent repair of congenital heart disease thirty years ago provides us with important information concerning the long-term results of the various types of operations. We now know that many defects such as secundum atrial septal defect, ventricular septal defect, pulmonary stenosis, patent ductus arteriosus, tetralogy of Fallot and coarctation of the aorta have an excellent prognosis following childhood repair. We know which defects may require another operation during adulthood. For example, patients with aortic stenosis who underwent aortic valvotomy or balloon valvuloplasty during childhood will eventually require aortic valve replacement. Patients who have had conduits placed between the right ventricle and the pulmonary artery usually require another operation ten or more years later because of conduit obstruction.

Some problems may not emerge for many years. The discovery of late problems can result in a change in management or even the type of operation performed in children today. For example, patients born with D-transposition of the great arteries are no longer treated with a Mustard or Senning operation during infancy as was the practice until the 1980s. Late problems after this operation in some adolescents and young adults led to the development of an alternative operation known as the arterial switch. This operation results in anatomic correction of D-transposition of the great arteries and to date has produced excellent long-term results.

Other important changes have occurred in the care of patients with congenital heart disease. The development of echocardiography in the 1980s and further refinements in this technique have revolutionized the management of patients with congenital heart disease. Echocardiography allows non-invasive diagnosis for nearly all forms of congenital heart disease. At major congenital heart disease centers, the use of echocardiography has dramatically decreased the need for diagnostic cardiac catheterization in patients with congenital heart disease. In addition, transesophageal echocardiography is now used in the operating room to assess the surgical repair at the conclusion of the operation.

When a cardiac catheterization is required, the procedure is safer and less traumatic today than it was in the past. In addition, recent interventions in the cardiac catheterization laboratory are decreasing the need for follow-up operations. For example, pulmonary artery narrowing can often be treated with balloon dilatation or pulmonary artery stenting. Aortic and pulmonary valve obstructions can usually be improved with balloon valvuloplasty. For patients with pulmonary stenosis, this procedure may eliminate the future need for cardiac surgery. For patients with aortic stenosis, the balloon valvuloplasty may delay for many years the need for aortic valve replacement.

Some forms of patent ductus arteriosus can now be closed with coils placed during a cardiac catheterization, instead of surgery. Devices have been developed to correct a very common form of congenital heart disease known as secundum atrial septal defect. Clinical trials are presently under way to determine the safety and effectiveness of this procedure. It is likely that this form of congenital heart disease will be treated in the future without cardiac surgery.

The care of the patient during and after cardiac surgery has steadily improved over the years. The length of hospitalization is much shorter now than in the past. Complicated cardiac operations can now be safely performed because of advances in both operative management and postoperative care. This includes better techniques for myocardial preservation during heart surgery, medications to decrease postoperative bleeding, and the development of potent intravenous medications to provide support for the heart muscle until it has recovered from the operation. For the most severe cases, mechanical assist devices are available in some centers that can provide temporary support when there is inadequate heart muscle function to maintain adequate perfusion to the body.

Are general heart-healthy practices (good diet, exercise) more important for someone with a congenital heart defect than for the average person?

Dr. Rosenbaum: Heart-healthy practices are recommended for all patients. Exercise and diet can reduce the incidence of coronary artery disease. While coronary artery disease is not an important issue in the pediatric population, we do want to modify risk factors that will predispose the patient to coronary obstructions later in life.

Certain types of congenital heart disease could be exacerbated by the development of coronary artery disease. For example, a patient with a single ventricle and Fontan repair could deteriorate if the ventricle were damaged by a myocardial infarction (heart attack). In addition, some patients with congenital heart disease have abnormal function of the right side of the heart. While patients may not experience any symptoms from this, we cannot predict how the right ventricle would perform if coronary artery obstruction developed and right ventricular function deteriorated further.

In general, is the life expectancy of a child with CHD shorter than that of someone who is born with a healthy heart?

Dr. Rosenbaum: The answer obviously depends on the type of congenital heart disease. For patients in whom surgical correction results in mild or no residual defects, such as those with secundum atrial septal defect, pulmonary stenosis, patent ductus arteriosus, coarctation of the aorta, ventricular septal defect, and tetralogy of Fallot, we would speculate that the life expectancy should be similar to that of people with a healthy heart.

In patients with some residual defects after heart surgery, such as a leak in the mitral valve following repair of a primum atrial septal defect or aortic regurgitation following valvuloplasty for aortic stenosis, we would also anticipate excellent longevity. However, some of these patients may eventually require another cardiac operation such as a valve replacement. When the correction for a particular form of congenital heart disease requires the use of artificial tubes or valves such as a conduit or homograft to connect the ventricle to the pulmonary artery, we can also anticipate additional operations in the future to replace an obstructed conduit or failing homograft.

In patients with a complex form of congenital heart disease known as a single ventricle, a Fontan operation often provides excellent palliation. The operation eliminates cyanosis and improves exercise capacity. Since very few patients with a Fontan operation have reached the age of forty, we do not yet have information concerning future problems later in adulthood. We have seen problems with arrhythmias and fluid retention in the young adults who underwent this procedure during the 1980s. As a result, the surgical procedure was subsequently modified in the hope that this will lead to a better long-term result.

In what ways does CHD impact the lives of your adult patients?

Dr. Rosenbaum: The impact of congenital heart disease on the lives of adults depends so much on their current cardiac status and any related problems. It is important to recognize that the adults whom we see today with congenital heart disease may have undergone surgery thirty years ago and their subsequent course bears little resemblance to the future population of adults who are currently children. Some of the repairs that we see in adults today are no longer even performed.

With these issues in mind, it can be said that most of the patients who have had successful cardiac surgery during childhood continue to do well as adults. Many are married and have successful careers. Patients who have had uncomplicated repairs are engaged in activities unencumbered by their cardiac problem. Patients who have residual defects require periodic follow-up and some may eventually require another operation during adulthood. I find it remarkable how well these patients have adjusted to the prospect of another future cardiac operation.

Exercise is an important issue for many young adults. Some patients have moderate valve abnormalities that can be monitored without cardiac surgery. However, these patients are often cautioned against participating in strenuous exercise. This type of limitation is sometimes very difficult for adolescents and young adults.

Some women will have concerns about the risks of pregnancy. While most women with adequately repaired congenital heart disease can tolerate the progressive increase in blood volume that occurs during pregnancy, some patients may experience problems as a pregnancy progresses. Couples are often concerned about the possibility of congenital heart disease in future offspring. While the incidence is somewhat higher than the general population, for most forms of congenital heart disease, the risk is approximately 5 percent.

Clearly, the advances in the treatment of congenital heart disease have been extraordinary.

FINDING THE INFORMATION YOU NEED

By Karen Klein, president, Adult Congenital Heart Association

I am twenty-seven years old, an ACHDer with uncorrected truncus arteriosus. I am a graduate student in library and information science, which has given me a special set of skills that have served me well as an adult with CHD. I want to share a few things I have learned so that you can be a more informed and empowered consumer of healthcare services. There are many resources you can use to conduct research on CHD. They can be divided into four categories: your doctors, libraries, the Internet, and other parents/patients.

YOUR DOCTORS

Your child's physicians are a valuable resource for information about CHD. They are most familiar with your child's case. It is their duty to help you understand issues such as your child's medical condition, procedures, and long-term prognosis. As such, finding the right doctors is vital. Your doctors should be knowledgeable about CHD, and you should be comfortable discussing your child's condition with them.

First, a word about training. Not all cardiologists are created equal. That is, there are several different kinds of cardiologists, and they receive different kinds of training. Pediatric cardiologists are trained, as the name indicates, to treat children. Since most patients with CHD are treated in childhood, pediatric cardiologists are trained to handle congenital anatomy. Adult cardiologists are primarily trained to handle patients with acquired heart disease, not CHD. As your child matures and begins to make the transition from adolescence to adulthood, you will eventually need to find an adult cardiologist. Doctors dealing with ACHDers should have a combination of pediatric and adult cardiology training to provide familiarity both with the structural/medical complications surrounding CHD, and adult issues such as sexuality and reproduction, complications related to aging, and issues related to adult lifestyles. Treating adults with CHD is not an official subspecialty in the United States, but there are practice guidelines published by the American College of Cardiology with regard to proper ACHD training. They are available on-line at http://www.acc.org/clinical/training/task9.htm or in print in the *Journal of the American College of Cardiology* (D. J. Skorton et al., 1995).

Some cardiologists who specialize in working with ACHDers have relationships with other doctors (e.g., primary care physicians, gynecologists, or dentists) who are accustomed to dealing with patients with CHD. If your child's cardiologist does not have such a list, or if for insurance or other reasons you cannot see those doctors, make sure that your other doctors are willing and able to communicate with the cardiologist and that they feel comfortable treating a patient with CHD. Ideally, you and all of your child's doctors should form a team to manage your child's care.

LIBRARIES

Just like cardiologists, not all libraries are the same. They vary in their collections by the intended audience. For example, a public library probably will not have as extensive a collection of medical journals as a medical school library. However, if the materials you seek are not held at your library, you can often procure them through interlibrary loan (ILL). There is sometimes a fee for ILL services, so it's a good idea to find out your library's policies before submitting requests. Some—but not all—medical school and hospital libraries have patient education centers, or will allow the public to use their collections.

If you are just starting to look for information, the reference desk is a good place to begin. The reference librarians are knowledgeable about the collection, as well as about some resources that might help you find what you are looking for. They also may be able to direct you to the best information for your level of knowledge. Often, a special reference section of the library holds basic reference books such as *Physician's Desk Reference* (a book that lists drugs, their effects, and side effects). The reference librarian can help you access databases such as Medline (a computerized index of medical articles). Remember, though, that the librarian is not a doctor. All he or she can do is guide you to the information, not interpret it for you. If you have questions about information you find, it is best to discuss them with your child's cardiologist.

THE INTERNET

The Internet offers a wealth of support and information on CHD in various forms. A listserv is a subscription-based (usually free) electronic message system. Subscribers send E-mail messages to a central address, whereupon each individual message is distributed to all subscribers of the list. People respond to messages posted to the listserv, and in this way discussions begin. There are listservs for both parents of children with CHD and adults with CHD.

Another resource to "meet" people and obtain information and support are on-line chat rooms, "places" on-line that computer users log onto to type messages back and forth to each other. There are Web-based chat rooms for parents and ACHDers.

A third, and probably the best-known, Internet resource is the Web. It's important to look at Web sites critically because of the glut of information that's out there. At present there are no universal professional standards to guide Web developers in documenting the sources of the information they present.

However, developers of health-related content can voluntarily adhere to the standards put forth by the Health On the Net Foundation (HONF). There are three important things to evaluate in beginning to determine the credibility of information found on the Web: the author, the institutional affiliation of the author, and the source of the information posted. All of these should be in plain view on the Web site.

Also consider the author's motives for posting the information. Is it simply information, or is the author trying to sell something?

There are different types of Web sites. Some are personal, some are commercial, some are by organizations, and others are by government agencies. The first step in evaluating a Web site is determining the authority of the site. Personal pages are often denoted by a "~," or the Web address will have a user name in it. An example would be http://www2.bc.edu/~kleinka/

Personal sites often feature a narrative of the person's experiences with CHD. There may also be "links," connections to other Web sites the Web site owner thinks are worth visiting, such as the American Heart Association Web site. The authors of personal sites are usually parents or patients, not medical professionals, so take any medical information they offer with a healthy dose of skepticism. Information on the site may be inaccurate. The links, however, may prove to be valuable, and in time you'll edit ("bookmark") your own collection of favorites.

Web sites published by nonprofit organizations usually have addresses that end in .org (e.g., http://www.achaheart.org), while commercial, for-profit organizations tend to use .com (e.g., http://www.aol.com). Even when the sponsoring organization is clearly identified, it's important to assess what type of organization it is. Just about anyone can start both nonprofit and for-profit corporations. Who is running the corporation? Is medical information on the site either written or reviewed by medical professionals? If not, or if you can't tell, then be cautious about what you read. Commercial sites are usually geared for selling some medicine, device, or treatment. Check to see if claims about the benefits of these products are backed up by citations or links to peer-reviewed medical literature.

Government published sites (web addresses containing .gov) are excellent sources of credible information. Government agencies such as the National Institutes of Health and the Centers for Disease Control and Prevention run a multitude of sites, some of which are meant for the average medical consumer, and some that are highly technical or specialized and difficult to wade through. At the very least these sites often include good links.

At any site, you'll want to know when it was last updated (this usually appears at the bottom of the home page). Return to the site often to see how frequently it is updated. A good site will not simply function as a wall of information. Look for phone numbers, E-mail addresses, and other contact information in case you have questions.

Finally, a site is only as good as it is usable. The usability of the site—how easy it is to access and use—is an important consideration. In general, a credible site will be easy to find, well organized, and easy to navigate. This also may be true of less credible sites, but a sloppy user-unfriendly site should raise a few red flags from the start. As with library materials, it is a good idea to discuss your concerns or questions about Web-based information with your child's physicians.

OTHER PARENTS/PATIENTS

Many parents and ACHDers feel lonely and isolated, and find great relief in making contact with other parents and ACHDers. Support networks and groups facilitate such contact and not infrequently lead to lasting friendships. Other parents and patients also can be resources for information about CHD and CHD specialists.

As I have learned, the ability to find information and enlist support are both invaluable skills for anyone coping with a lifelong illness.

MUTUAL SUPPORT:
CREATING COMMUNITY ON-LINE
By Diane C. Clapp, founder and facilitator, AOL ACHD chat

I am a forty-one-year-old ACHDer with tricuspid atresia and the founder of a weekly on-line chat for ACHDers on America Online (AOL). I want to share with you the story about how I started this chat, which is just one example of how to form a support community.

In July 1996 I signed up for an Internet service not only to find information about my specific type of CHD but also with the hope of finding other adults with the same or similar health problems. The first places I looked once I got on-line were the health bulletin boards and a listing for congenital heart defects. Most of the postings were from parents of children with CHD, but there were one or two messages from ACHDers. In responding to one of these postings, I discovered a fellow ACHDer who not only shared the same doctor but also the same cardiac anatomy. I had never met anyone "like me" before.

As I continued to explore the Internet for information about CHD I soon discovered two other important means of support. First, in August 1996 I found a mutual support "chat" for cardiac patients. Second, in December I came upon the ACHD listserv.

In the cardiac chat I soon recognized a big difference between the

concerns of someone with congenital heart defects and those of someone with acquired heart disease. The cardiac chat discussions centered largely around stories about heart attacks and treatment, high
blood pressure, and cholesterol, especially ways to control them
through diet and exercise. Diet and exercise will not change a congenital heart defect. One night in the chat I asked about a surgical procedure I'd been through recently. When no one knew what I was
talking about I realized that we ACHDers needed our own chat.

To start a new chat area within my Internet service provider's
health network, I had to meet two criteria. One, I had to be familiar
with and have firsthand knowledge of the topic. (Having CHD helped
meet this criterion.) Two, there had to be at least fifteen individuals interested in participating in a weekly chat.

I first posted a message on the bulletin board and the adult CHD
listserv asking if there were any other ACHDers who would be interested in attending an on-line support group/chat. I got quite a few
responses to my posting, including one from a woman in Texas who
would later become my cofacilitator. After weeks of planning and
debate, we decided that the best day and time for the chat was on Sat-
urdays at 11:00 P.M. EST. We chose Saturday because of the large number of college students who had responded to my initial posting, and
11:00 P.M. so we could accommodate people in all U.S. time zones.

On the first Saturday night of April 1997, the unofficial ACHD chat
started up as a private chat. Nine ACHDers joined that night for an
open discussion about CHD. I continued posting notices about the
chat on the ACHD bulletin board and sending E-mails to any ACHDers
I found on-line. I would tell them about the group and ask them if they
would like to join us. Soon we had the required fifteen participants.

By midsummer I felt it was time to move the chat to a location on
the Internet that would offer greater visibility and provide easier access. The current "location" was difficult for new ACHDers to find, because they had to know in advance that we existed. In our new place,
we could be found more easily through a special listing of health-
related topics and discussions.

In late summer I wrote to AOL, telling them that we had reached
the required attendance. I requested the same day and time. We were
assigned to what was known then as the personal empowerment
room. On October 4, 1997, the official ACHD chat began on the health
network. That night's topic was "Fall routine: Do you take longer than
most to adjust to a new routine?" Fourteen people attended.

One of my most challenging duties as the facilitator is trying to create fresh and interesting topics that pertain to growing up and living with CHD as an adult. Some of those topics have been:

- Tell your favorite hospital story
- How did your CHD affect your siblings?
- Insurance—life and health
- Health proxies and consent forms

I also maintain a list of screen names for the monthly mailings and try to keep track of each person's CHD diagnosis.

Unless you have grown up with a birth defect or any other childhood abnormality, it's hard to understand the emotional and psychological aspects of it. Even with tremendous family support, you can still feel alone. You're not only dealing with the same issues as any other child—homework, trying to figure out math—but also putting up with the bullies who harass you about your blue lips and blue fingernails. And there's the prejudice of teachers and other people who fear you will pass out—or worse. Cycles of clinic appointments, hospital stays, and frequent diagnostic procedures and tests run the gamut from annoying to grueling, and further remind you that you're different. You sense the worry and concern of your family and friends, and you worry about them worrying about you. Even with family, friends, doctors, and nurses around you and helping you, you are the one who is actually going through these things.

As an adult you have other concerns, such as when and how to explain your CHD to someone you're dating, convincing someone that you're capable of doing the job they are hiring you for despite your heart defect, and wondering if you'll be able to get that much-needed health insurance. With marriage, you wonder if you'll be able to have children and how your CHD will affect your spouse and your children.

I have watched the chat group grow from being a kinship of adults with a mutual rarity into a family of very close friends. We worry a lot about each other, and when we haven't heard from someone in a while we write or call to see if that person is okay. We ask each other how our doctors' appointments went. We have even convinced people to call a doctor or go to the ER when they weren't feeling well.

In August 1997 my cofacilitator was going to be in the Boston area. This gave us the chance to meet for the first time. We invited other members to join us in a small pizza party. Now we are trying to make this an annual ACHD gathering.

On occasion I get discouraged about running the chat due to the difficulty of coming up with topics and keeping up the attendance. I even wonder whether it is doing any good. Then I get notes from new people who participated in a recent chat, saying not only how much they enjoyed the chat but also how they feel relieved to finally be able to find and talk to others who have been through the same things.

They often say, "Wow, I thought I was the only one."

Then I remember how I felt and why I started the chat.

GLOSSARY

amniocentisis. A test where a needle is used to extract fluid from the amniotic sac that surrounds a fetus. The results of this test can indicate a fetal abnormality.

anemia. Low blood count.

anesthesia. A drug or gas that produces a partial or total loss of the sense of pain, temperature, touch, etc.

angiocardiography. The science of injecting contrast media (dye) into the heart and blood vessels to obtain high-quality X-ray motion pictures. It is performed during cardiac catheterization.

anticoagulate. To thin, as in blood.

aorta. Main blood vessel from the heart to the body.

arrhythmia. An irregularity of the heart rate or rhythm.

artery. A tube that carries blood from the heart to all the other parts of the body.

atresia. Absence or abnormal constriction of any natural passage of the body.

atrium. Either of two sections in the top part of the heart that receives blood from the veins.

bradycardia. An abnormally slow heart rate.

cardiologist. A doctor who is trained to take care of the heart.

cardiopulmonary bypass. Surgery using the heart/lung machine.

catheter. A very skinny, hollow tube, often used to diagnose and treat heart defects.

chromosomes. A part of the cell that carries the genes that give living things their characteristics.

coil embolization. A procedure in which a tiny metal coil is placed inside an unwanted blood vessel to close it off.

coronary. Related to the heart.

cyanosis. Blueness.

ductus arteriosus. Muscular tube that connects the aorta (vessel to the body) and the pulmonary artery (vessel to the lungs).

diuretic. Something that increases the urinary discharge.

echocardiogram (echo). A test using sound waves (ultrasound) to study the structure of the heart.

electrocardiogram (EKG). A test that records the electrical activity of the heart.

endocarditis. An infection of the inner lining of the heart.

fetal echocardiogram. An ultrasound of the baby's heart while it is still in the mother's womb.

fetus. The offspring in the womb, from the end of the third month of pregnancy until birth.

hypothermia. Below normal body temperature.

in utero. Inside a mother's womb.

magnetic resonance imaging. A series of pictures of the heart and blood vessels made with a large magnet and computer processing.

murmur. A noise that can be heard only with a stethoscope.

myocarditis. An inflammation of the heart muscle.

palliation. A procedure that lessens the pain or severity of the defect, without curing it.

pericardium. The sac that surrounds the heart.

prophylaxis. The prevention of disease.

pulmonary. To do with the lungs.

pulmonary artery. Blood vessel that takes blood to the lungs.

regurgitation. Leaking.

septum. A dividing wall.

shunt. Any connection between the systemic (aortic) circulation and the pulmonary (lung) circulation.

sonogram/ultrasound. A test using sound waves to create pictures of the structure of the fetus.

stenosis. A narrowing of a passage, duct, or opening.

stent. A wire mesh tube used to prop open an artery.

syncope. A fainting or loss of consciousness.

tachycardia. An abnormally fast heart rate.

teratogen. Any environmental agent that produces or increases the likelihood of fetal harm.

vein. A vessel through which blood is carried back to the heart from other parts of the body.

ventilator. A breathing machine. Also called a respirator.

ventricle. Either one of the two lower chambers of the heart. The ventricles receive blood from the atria and pump it to the arteries.

RESOURCES
∽

WE ARE HAPPY to say that our resource list only scratches the surface of what's out there today. The CHD community has certainly come a long way since our children were diagnosed. Incredible support and plenty of information is there if you look. In addition to the resources we list, we encourage you to seek out local support groups. You can find them through your hospital or pediatric cardiologist and from some of the comprehensive Web sites.

Information and Support

CHASER: Congenital Heart Anomalies, Support, Education and Resources, Inc.

CHASER is a national organization meeting the needs and addressing the concerns of families of children with CHD through one-on-one support, information, resources, and advocacy.

CHASER
2112 North Wilkins Road
Swanton, OH 43558
Phone: (419) 825-5575
Fax: (419) 825-2880
E-mail: CHASER@compuserve.com
www.csun.edu/~hfmth006/chaser/

The Congenital Heart Disease Resource Page

This Web site, maintained by Sheri Berger, should be one of your first stops in your Internet search. It provides comprehensive information on congenital heart defects, as well as links to many other sites.

www.bamdad.com/sheri/

Congenital Heart Information Network (C.H.I.N.)

"Our goal is to provide information, support, and resources to families of children with congenital and acquired heart disease, adults with CHD, and the professionals who work with them." This site is a gateway to a myriad of resources and on-line support groups.

Congenital Heart Information Network
1561 Clark Drive
Yardley, PA 19067
Phone: (215) 493-3068
E-mail: mb@tchin.org (Mona Barmash)
www.tchin.org

PDHeart

PDHeart is an E-mail forum for people with CHD, their families, and other concerned individuals to share information and experiences, and to provide support. PDHeart currently has over 800 members from many countries around the world. To subscribe to the mailing list, go to www.tchin. org or send E-mail to pdheart-on@tchin.org.

The Congenital Heart Disease Webring

This Webring is a growing collection of Web sites about congenital heart defects that are all linked together. This is a wonderful resource if you're interested in reading personal stories and viewing photos of kids with CHD, both in and out of the hospital.

www.adventureangling.com/chd/webring.htm

Yahoo—Congenital Heart Defect Support

This group is about raising and supporting people with congenital heart defects. There is a chat room and you can post messages to the site.

clubs.yahoo.com/clubs/congenitalheartdefectsupport

Yahoo—Congenital Heart Defect Grandparents Support

This Web site's goal is to provide support, friendship and a common meeting place for grandparents of children with CHD.

clubs.yahoo.com/clubs/grandparentsofchd

Canadian Adult Congenital Heart (CACH) Network

Comprehensive care and information for adult patients with congenital heart disease and their care providers.

www.cachnet.org

Kids With Heart (KWH)

A nonprofit, volunteer organization established to educate and enhance the lives of children and their loved ones about heart defects or acquired heart disease, KWH runs a support group for families. Call for a registration form about parent matching and adult matching. You can be matched up with others based on diagnosis, location or hospital.

Michelle L. Rintamaki
1578 Careful Drive
Green Bay, WI 54304
E-mail: stempa@execpc.com
Phone: 1-800-538-5390
www.execpc.com/~kdswhrt

The Heart Center Encyclopedia

This informational Web site is a great resource for families of children with CHD. Prepared by doctors at the Children's Hospital Medical Center of Cincinnati, it addresses many questions about CHD and offers basic information about the heart, different types of defects, and different types of treatments. You'll also find color and animated pictures of the defects.

www.cincinnatichildrens.org/heartcenter/encyclopedia/

Grown-Up Congenital Heart Patients' Association (GUCH)

Run by and for teenagers and adults with congenital heart disease, GUCH seeks to support and enable normal living and to educate society about the needs and gifts of this new group of people who have survived as a result of advances in cardiac medicine.

Judy Shedden (National Coordinator)
Beech Cottage
26A Quarry Road
Winchester SO23 0JG
England

Help line: (+44) (0) 800 854759
Fax: (+44) (0) 1962 841635
E-mail: judy@guch.demon.co.uk (Judy Shedden)
www.guch.demon.co.uk

Children's Heart Society

A nonprofit, nongovernment-funded charitable organization that is totally operated by volunteers and that supports families of children with heart disease.

Box 52088, Garneau Postal Outlet
Edmonton, AB T6G 2T5
Canada
Phone: (403) 454-7665
CHS pager: (403) 497-9077
Toll-free: (800) CHS-9404
E-mail: ch@childrensheart.org
www.childrensheart.org/

Left Heart Matters

This group has a number of objectives, which include raising the public and medical profession's awareness of hypoplastic left heart syndrome and providing support and advice to parents who have a child with a hypoplastic left heart.

Left Heart Matters
c/o Deb Rahman or Sister Suzie Hutchison
24 Calthorpe Road
Edgbaston
West Midlands, United Kingdom B15 1RP
Phone: 0121 455 8982
Fax: 0121 455 8983
E-mail: info@lhm.org.uk
www.lhm.org.uk

Adult Congenital Heart Association

At press time, this group was planning its second annual conference. Their comprehensive Web site for adults with CHD includes a link to their newsletter, The Laurel Wreath. They also sponsor a weekly chat on AOL.

ACHA
c/o Karen Klein
273 Perham Street
West Roxbury, MA 02132
Phone: (617) 325-1191
E-mail: info@achaheart.org

The Laurel Wreath
c/o Diane Clapp
308 Matfield Street
West Bridgewater, MA 02379
E-mail: dcc8@aol.com

Research Organizations

The Heart of a Child Foundation

Funds research to find the root causes of congenital heart defects and to improve the care and treatment of children born with these defects.

Rashida and Raghu Mendu
26710 Fond Du Lac Road
Rancho Palos Verdes, CA 90275
Phone: (310) 375-6617
Fax: (310) 388-5917
www.heartofachild.org

Children's Cardiac Research

Benefits pediatric cardiology research at the University of Miami and elsewhere, and provides support, information, and assistance to families of children with congenital and acquired heart defects.

Children's Cardiac Research Foundation, Inc.
P.O. Box 77-2801
Coral Springs, FL 33077
Phone: (954) 753-0711 or (800) 436-6499
E-mail: Bgccrf@aol.com
www.childsheart.com

Summer Camps

Camp Del Corazon, Inc.

This 501(c) nonprofit corporation provides, free of charge, a summer camp for children with heart disease. All proceeds are spent entirely on the camp.

5655 Halbrent Avenue, #10
Van Nuys, CA 91411
Phone: (818) 901-0323
Fax: (818) 901-0323
E-mail: info@campdelcorazon.org
www.campdelcorazon.org

Camp Bon Coeur

Camp "Good Heart" is a nonprofit two-week residential camp for children with acquired or congenital heart defects.

Camp Bon Coeur
A Rehabilitative Cardiac Camp
P.O. Box 53765
Lafayette, LA 70505
Phone: (318) 233-8437
E-mail: Campbonc@net-connect.net
www.heartcamp.com

Camp Braveheart

Camp Braveheart's mission is to create a positive life experience for all children through a camping program that promotes self-esteem, socialization among peers, support from other families dealing with complex heart defects, and so much fun.

3495 Brittany Way
Kennesaw, GA 30152
Phone: (888) 988-9979 or (770) 919-2775
E-mail: campbraveheart@geocities.com
www.geocities.com/EnchantedForest/Tower/9877

Boggy Creek Hole In the Wall Gang Camp

Hole in the Wall Gang camps were founded by Paul Newman, General H. Norman Schwarzkopf and others. Boggy Creek, located on 232 acres 40 minutes north of Orlando, is an extension of the original camp in Ashford, Connecticut. The camp hosts family weekends in the spring and kids-only weeks in the summer. Activities include swimming, boating, arts and crafts, dancing, and much more. Since the camp serves children with all different chronic illnesses, check to find out the dates reserved for CHD kids.

30500 Brantley Branch Road
Eustis, FL 32736
Phone: (352) 483-4200
Fax: (352) 483-0358
E-mail: info@boggycreek.org
www.boggycreek.org

Hope with Heart

A week-long camp that allows children with heart conditions to connect with other children who have similar health issues, to realize that they are not alone and to enjoy their childhood as every child should.

P.O. Box 618
Hewitt, NJ 07421
Phone: (973) 728-3854
E-mail: hopewithheart@hotmail.com
www.hopewithheart.com

The Edward Madden Memorial Open Hearts Camp

Situated on 400 acres of rolling hills in the Berkshire Mountains of Massachusetts, the Madden Camp is a summer retreat where children with CHD can enjoy outdoor sports and recreational activities. The camp program is specifically tailored to the needs of children who have recovered from open-heart or heart transplant surgery, including those children who may previously have been unable to enjoy sports and other activities that most kids take for granted. Attending Madden Camp is free. Parents are responsible only for the cost of transportation to and from camp.

Louise Cowin, Director
250 Monument Valley Road
Great Barrington, MA 02130
Phone: (888) 611-1113 (winter) or (413) 528-2229 (summer)
E-mail: info@openheartscamp.com
www.openheartscamp.com

Transplant Information

National Transplant Assistance Fund (NTAF)

NTAF is a not-for-profit resource serving all organ and tissue transplant patients, their families, and the professional community that treats them. NTAF also provides services for patients with catastrophic injury. They provide fund-raising expertise for patients raising money for uninsured medically related expenses, $1000 grants for eligible patients, and education on organ/tissue donation.

Suite 230
3475 West Chester Pike
Newtown Square, PA 19073
Phone: (800) 642-8399 or (610) 353-9684
Fax: (610) 353-1616
E-mail: NTAF@transplantfund.org
www.transplantfund.org

American Share Foundation

Offers a Web site with information, but not medical advice, for the transplant community, including patients, families, caregivers, healthcare professionals, support networks, and the general public.

John S. Abbott, Founder of American Share Foundation & ASCOT
E-mail: jabbott@ntx.com (John Abbott)
web742d8.ntx.net/viewer.html

Children's Helpers Educating, Reassuring and Uniting by Sharing (CHERUBS)

A nonprofit organization whose primary objective is to save the lives of children who are waiting for organ transplants.

CHERUBS
P.O. Box 2292
North Bend, WA 98045
E-mail: sandyman@cherubs.org
www.cherubs.org/index.html

Transplant Recipients International Organization, Inc. (TRIO)

An international independent not-for-profit organization committed to improving the quality of life of transplant candidates, recipients, their families, and donor families. Promotes donor awareness, support, education, and advocacy.

1000 16th Street, NW, Suite 602
Washington, DC 20036-5705
Phone: (800) TRIO-386 or (202) 293-0980
Fax: (202) 293-0973
E-mail: trio@mindspring.com
www.primenet.com/~trio/

Air Transport Agencies

The following is a list of agencies that can be called to help provide air transportation to and from hospitals and appointments:*

American Airlines

(Miles for Kids in Need). This is a once-a-lifetime service for children up to eighteen years old.
Phone: (817) 963-8118

Delta Airlines

Skywish Program. This program is a combined effort of The United Way and Delta Airlines to help people with life-threatening illnesses travel to and from their appointments. The patient plus one person may fly free, round trip, once every six months. It takes five days to process the request.
Phone: (800) 892-2757, ext. 285

National Patient Air Transportation Helpline

Call or log on for information and referrals to sources of help available through the Angel Flight America Network.
Phone: (800) 296-1217
http://www.npath.org/

The following are names of discount ticket agencies provided by The United Way:
TFI of New York: (800) 745-8000
Travel Bargains: (800) 247-3273
Cheaptickets: (800) 377-1000

*This information is correct, to our knowledge, as of publication. Unfortunately, it's possible the information has changed since publication.

OTHER BOOKS OF INTEREST
∞

Many of these books are available through the Internet or at your local bookstore or library.

Books for Teaching Children about the Body

Nigel Nelson, *Looking Into My Body* (New York: Reader's Digest Children's Books, 1995).

Simple, scientifically correct illustrations on transparent plastic. The text is short and easy to read and understand. Includes a nice colorful drawing of the heart. Recommended for ages 4 to 8.

Steve Parker, *How The Body Works* (Pleasantville, N.Y.: Reader's Digest, 1994).

Encourages children to learn by discovery with experiments to help them understand the body's functions. The section on the heart includes a make-your-own stethoscope activity, an EKG diagram, and more. Aimed at ages 8 to 14.

Richard Platt, *Stephen Biesty's Incredible Body: Meet the Teams that Make the Body Work* (New York: DK Publishing, 1998).

Uses the perspective of tiny people traveling through a man's body to present its various systems and organs. Huge and detailed illustrations.

Melanie and Chris Rice, *My First Body Book* (New York: DK Publishing, 2001).

See-through pages let you peer inside the human body layer by layer. Simple, clear explanations accompanied by bold, colorful illustrations, photos, and activities make this book attractive to younger children. Recommended for ages 4 to 8.

Seymour Simon, *The Heart: Our Circulatory System* (New York: Mulberry Books, 1996).

This book includes incredible computer-enhanced graphic images of a beating heart in action, red blood cells pushing through tiny capillaries, and more. In a subtle and direct way, the author takes the reader on a journey and shows the heart and circulatory system to be a wondrous thing. Appropriate for ages 4 to 14.

Kate Barnes and Steve Weston, *How It Works—The Human Body*, (New York: Barnes and Noble Books, 1997).

This book contains wonderful clear and simple illustrations and explanations of how the heart works. Appropriate for ages 4 to 14.

Congenital Heart Disease

Catherine Neill, M.D., Edward Clark, M.D., and Carleen Clark, R.N., *The Heart of a Child* (Baltimore: Johns Hopkins University Press, 2001).

An overview of congenital heart disease and the most common methods of treatment, including descriptions of defects both directly and indirectly associated with CHD, as well as many illustrations. Several case studies help the reader relate to each situation. This book is easy to read and each term is clearly defined.

Mary Kleinman, *Congenital Heart Disease (What the Doctor Didn't Tell You about)* (Salt Lake City: Northwest Publishing, 1993).

A general book about congenital heart disease and its impact on children and families. Kleinman explains thirty defects and provides detailed illustrations. Of particular interest is the chapter titled "A Medical Introduction," with its emphasis on embryology and the development of the human heart. A thorough glossary of medical terms and concise explanations of diagnostic and surgical procedures round out this valuable resource for parents.

Anna Marie Jaworski, *Hypoplastic Left Heart Syndrome: A Handbook for Parents* (Temple, Tex.: Baby Hearts Press, 1995).

Anna Jaworski and her husband, Frank Jaworski, R.N., have put together a valuable resource for parents of children with hypoplastic left heart syndrome, their own son being one of these children. Jaworski first takes you through her personal experiences and emotions, then goes on to discuss the different options parents must consider: surgery, transplantation, or doing nothing. The book also details the different procedures, what to expect before and after surgery, what social services are available, and illustrates the defects and corrective procedures. This book is a must for any parent needing to make the difficult decisions about the care of their HLHS child.

Maryann Anglim and Walter Allan, *Kara Mia* (Bath, Maine: Seahorse Press, 1997).

Describes the personal and professional saga of a fourteen-year-old girl who collapses at track practice from Long QT syndrome and suffers anoxic brain injury. This true story provides a unique insight into the thoughts and feelings of her family and her physician as they struggle to understand her condition and rehabilitate her. *Kara Mia* chronicles all the difficult steps along the way, from Kara's resuscitation, prolonged hospital stay, and diagnosis of Long QT syndrome to her continuing rehabilitation outside the hospital. It is a story of love and support, tears and laughter. Black-and-white photographs show Kara with family, friends, and medical staff as she improves. A glossary and bibliography are included.

Surgery and the Hospital

Claire Ciliotta and Carole Livingston, *Why Am I Going to the Hospital?: A Helpful Guide to a New Experience*, illustrated by Dick Wilson (Secaucus, N.J.: Lyle Stuart, 1981).

Introduces children to some of the sights and action in a hospital and illustrates the "star" treatment they can expect to help them get well. It speaks beautifully to a child about to be hospitalized.

Amy Moses, *At the Hospital* (Chanhassen, Minn.: The Child's World, 1998).

Simple text and photos present a hospital, its people, and its objects.

Nancy Keene and Rachel Prentice, *Your Child In the Hospital: A Practical Guide for Parents* (Sebastopol, Calif.: O'Reilly, 1997).

Helps parents prepare their child physically and emotionally for the trip to the hospital.

Sara Bonnett Stein, photographs by Doris Pinney, *A Hospital Story: An Open Family Book for Parents and Children Together* (New York: Walker, 1974).

This unique presentation of a hospital visit creates a shared experience for adult and child. There is separate text for adults and for children, giving each the tools they need to cope with a hospital visit.

Seymour Reito, *Some Busy Hospital*, illustrated by Carolyn Bracken, (New York: Golden Books, 1985).

Simple text describes the special care that doctors and nurses give their patients, and the important work of all the other people on the staff. Lively, appealing illustrations convey a sense of warmth and activity. All in all, a reassuring introduction to the hospital.

Fred Rogers, *Going to the Hospital* (New York: Putnam and Grosset Group, 1988).

TV's Mr. Rogers gives children a very general overview of going to the hospital.

Anne Civardi and Stephen Cartwright, *Going to the Hospital* (London: Usborne, 1995).

Another general picture of the hospital for children.

Deborah Hautzig, *A Visit to the Sesame Street Hospital*, illustrated by Joe Mathieu (New York: Random House, 1985).

Grover, Ernie, and Bert take a tour of the hospital to prepare for Grover's tonsillectomy.

James Howe, *The Hospital Book* (New York: Beech Tree Books, 1994).

An excellent resource for children age four or over. Topics include general information about the hospital environment, descriptions of hospital personnel and their various duties, routine tests and procedures, the operating room, etc. Many black-and-white photographs add to this realistic view of what the child is likely to encounter.

James Howe, *A Night Without Stars* (Ormond Beach, Fla.: Camelot, 1993).

A heartwarming story about a special friendship that develops between two hospitalized children: a young girl scheduled for surgical repair of a VSD, and a preadolescent burn patient. Although the medical information is dated, the book chronicles the psychological experience of a child awaiting heart surgery in a realistic fashion. Recommended for ages nine through adult. Great family reading!

Jean Clabough, R.N., *Matty's Heart: A Child's and Parent's Guide to Open-Heart Surgery* (Alethia Publishing, 1995).

The story of Matthew Lewis told by the character Mr. Pump. Mr. Pump takes you from the time Matty was born and diagnosed through his doctor's office visits and the surgery, covering different tests (e.g., EKGs and echocardiograms) as well as what to expect before and after surgery. It is strongly suggested that you review the book first yourself and then read and discuss it with your child. It may well help allay your young one's fears, but you know your child best and what he or she can process.

Also see the accompanying coloring book, *Matty's Heart Cath.*

Siblings

Mary Thompson, *My Brother Matthew* (Bethesda, Md.: Woodbine House, 1992).

An uplifting book about a boy whose little brother is born with special needs. The baby is in the ICU at the hospital, comes home, and needs therapies and a lot of his parents' attention.

Donald Meyer, ed., *Views from Our Shoes: Growing Up with a Brother or Sister with Special Needs* (Bethesda, Md.: Woodbine House, 1997).

A collection of essays by children with siblings who have special needs. This book covers a variety of disabilities, but it deals with many issues that are universal when one child in the house is sick.

Pat Lowery Collins, *Waiting for Baby Joe* (Morton Grove, Ill.: Albert Whitman, 1990).

Realistic text and photographs chronicle the effect of Baby Joe's premature birth on young Missy and her family.

Joeri and Piet Breebaart, *When I Die Will I Get Better?* (New York: Peter Bedrick Books, 1993).

This book deals with the death of a sibling using the story of two brothers, Joe and Fred Rabbit.

Debra J. Lobato, *Brothers, Sisters, and Special Needs: Information and Activities for Helping Young Siblings of Children with Chronic Illnesses and Developmental Disabilities* (Baltimore: Paul H. Brookes, 1990).

Dr. Lobato thoroughly examines the relationships between siblings when one has a chronic disease and the other does not. She discusses psychological adjustments and considers why some siblings adjust better than others. Activities help siblings get to know their personal strengths and recognize positive characteristics of their brother or sister.

Debbie Duncan, Illustrations by Nina Ollikainen, M.D., *When Molly Was in the Hospital: A Book for Brothers and Sisters of Hospitalized Children* (Windsor, Calif.: Rayve Productions, 1994).

This beautifully illustrated storybook centers on a young girl whose sister becomes ill and is hospitalized for surgery. It's an honest portrayal of the child's feelings and the family's experience throughout the events of the sibling's illness, hospitalization, and recovery. Recommended for ages five to ten.

Down Syndrome

Karen Stray-Gunderson, ed., *Babies with Down Syndrome: A New Parents' Guide* (Bethesda, Md.: Woodbine House, 1995).

A wonderful, optimistic guide to Down syndrome that combines medical facts with encouragement from other parents.

Coping with Illness

Jill Krementz, ed., *How It Feels to Fight for Your Life* (New York: Little, Brown, 1989).

Fourteen children tell how they battle pain, uncertainty, and the changes brought about in their lives by serious illness such as heart defects, cancer, severe burns, asthma, and kidney failure.

Norma Simon, *Why Am I Different?*, illustrated by Dora Leader (Morton Grove, Ill.: Albert Whitman, 1976).

This children's book does not deal directly with disease, but with differences among people in general.

Kelly Huegel, *Young People and Chronic Illness* (Minneapolis: Free Spirit, 1998).

A helpful guide to coping with assorted illnesses, including CHD. This book is written for kids and is especially good for older children.

Suzanne LeVert, *Your Child and Health Care: A Dollars and Sense Guide for Families with Special Needs* (Baltimore: Paul H. Brookes, 1994).

A valuable resource guide for families with children who have special health care needs and the professionals who work with them. This book points to hundreds of resources for financial assistance, civil rights, educational services, and support organizations, and includes important guidelines for appealing denied health insurance claims, and practical advice on securing services for children.

Judith Loseff Lavin, *Special Kids Need Special Parents* (New York: Berkely Publishing Group, 2001).

A comprehensive resource for parents of children with special needs. Chapters deal with the point of view of the parent, the child, and other siblings. This book covers physical, emotional, and behavioral topics and is relevant for many disabilities and many different age groups.

VIDEOS

∽

Sesame Street Visits the Hospital

Realistic without being frightening. Unfortunately, it is currently out of print. You may be able to find it in a library or on the Internet.

The Adventures of Curious George

This irresistible video includes a segment on George's trip to the hospital.

INDEX

ABOUT THE AUTHORS

Gerri Freid Kramer is a vice president and a senior writer/producer for DWJ Television, a broadcast public relations company. She telecommutes full time from her home in Tampa, Florida, where she lives with her husband, Jeff Kramer, and her sons, Ethan and Max. Gerri graduated from Duke University, where Max later underwent successful surgery for a heart defect when he was three and a half weeks old.

Shari Maurer spent six years at the Children's Television Workshop working on international productions of *Sesame Street*. She graduated from Duke University and received an M.F.A. in Dramatic Writing from New York University. Shari lives in New City, New York, with her husband, Dr. Mathew Maurer, a cardiologist at Columbia University/New York Presbyterian Hospital, and their three children, Elisabeth, Joshua, and Eric. Elisabeth was born with tetralogy of Fallot, which was repaired when she was fourteen months old.